A NEW FIGHTING CHANCE
SILVER SOLUTION

FOURTH EDITION

A Quantum Leap in Silver Technology:

How molecular structuring safely
destroys bacteria, viruses and yeast.

GORDON PEDERSEN

Ph.D., N.D., FAPWCA, FAARM, Board Certified
Anti-Aging and Regenerative Medicine

To Order Additional Copies Please Call: 801.923.4352 or visit Amazon.com, DrGoPed.com or SilverHealthInstitute.com.

Table of Contents

What Is This New Structured Silver?

Silver is today where penicillin was 80 years ago, but it won't have penicillin's problems and won't require a prescription. It comes in many forms, the most popular of which are liquid and gel.

Liquid silver is a remarkably simple antimicrobial solution. It is composed of 0.001% pure metallic silver and 99.999% pure water.

The new structured silver is also alkaline. And that's it. All other silver liquids are acidic. The alkaline structured silvers are manufactured with high intensity electromagnetic pulses at a frequency that produces an alkaline charge. This is great for the body because it is designed to work in conjunction with the human body and can be taken every day. While the acidic forms of silver are good for temporary relief, their acidic nature makes it more difficult on your body to take on a regular basis.

Although it may have a faint metallic or medicine-like taste to it, the new silver is a clear liquid that looks and smells like water. That's because it is 99.999% water. Yet it is changing the way we think of preventive medicine.

It is safe enough to self-administer and yet destroys the cause of the most dangerous diseases known to humanity. It is changing the way we prevent disease and defend ourselves against contagious diseases because it works even when we don't know what the disease is.

It destroys the cause of disease and does so with a greater spectrum of activity than any antibiotic, making it a natural alternative to antibiotics. Yet, unlike most pharmaceutical products, it has no side effects.

The silver particles have specific and unique characteristics, including a specific size, a specific electron configuration, a specific magnetic resonance, a specific pH, a specific magnetic signature, and a specific structuring effect on the water molecules. Silver technology has made huge improvements over the old-style colloidal silvers of 100 years ago.

The resulting combination of silver and water has some very unusual properties. Some of these effects are best understood through the lens of physics as opposed to chemistry. Considering that most people view their health through the lens of biochemistry, the effectiveness of this new silver can catch people by surprise.

Specifically, the newest and most effective structured silver liquids can be identified by these characteristics:

· 10–30 ppm silver in water
· A mild alkaline pH (7.0 to 7.6 pH)
· Molecular structuring (structured water)
· Magnetic properties
· Quality control that is vastly improved over old-style silvers

If you are using a silver liquid that is acidic, ionic, or does not use structured water, you are not using the latest and most effective products.

The gel form of silver contains a similar combination of silver and water, but has also been pH-adjusted so that it is ideal for topical use. It has been made with maximum safety and purity in mind. Unlike many cosmetic products that contain carcinogens, pesticides, reproductive toxins, and hormone disruptors, this new gel does not. With specific reference to the David Suzuki Foundation's "Dirty Dozen" list of substances to avoid in cosmetic products, newer silver gels do not contain:

· BHA or BHT (preservatives that may cause cancer and endocrine disruption)
· Coal tar dyes; p-phenylenediamine (artificial colors with heavy metals and cancer-causing potential)
· DEA, MEA, and TEA (eg. triethanolamine)
· Bibutyl phthalate
· Formaldehydes
· Parabens
· Parfum
· PEGs (eg. polyethylene glycol)
· Petroatum

- Siloxanes
- Sodium laureth sulfate
- Triclosan

If you are using a silver gel that contains parfum, TEA, or other substances listed above, you are NOT using the latest and best products.

In summary, silver is an unusual combination of silver and water that safely kills pathogens. It comes in a newly perfected structured form that offers outstanding benefits without side effects or harmful chemicals.

It might save your life or the lives of people you love.

In homeopathic medicine the energy and dilution determine the effectiveness of the solution. Structured Silver has an energy that is homeopathic. This silver energy

Silver History

Silver has been used as medicine and a preservative by many cultures throughout history. Ancient Greeks used silver vessels for water purification. Pioneers trekking across the American west used it to keep their water safe and prevent dysentery, colds, and flu; they actually put silver dollars in their milk containers and wooden water casks to retard the growth of bacteria. Settlers in the Australian outback suspended silverware in their water tanks to retard spoilage. People in India still wrap some food and candies in a thin silver foil to prevent spoilage, which is then literally consumed along with the food.

Medicinal silver compounds were developed in the late 1800's and there was widespread use of silver compounds and colloids (small particles dispersed in water) prior to 1930. By 1940 there were approximately 48 different silver compounds marketed and used to treat virtually every infectious disease. These were available in oral, injectable, and topical forms. They carried such names as: Albargin, Novargan, Proganol, and Silvol.[1]

Since 1973, silver has been shown to have topical activity against 22 bacterial species (643 isolates), including gram-positive and gram-negative bacteria.[2] Ongoing research into the effect and properties of silver continues around the world.

Currently, silver water purification filters are used by organizations that include international airliners and NASA. Increasing numbers of Americans use silver in their fabrics, appliances, and home water filters. Electrical ionization units are being used in swimming pool water to help sanitize the water without the harsh effects of chlorine. Silver is also found in many applications within our hospitals, from needles to bandages to disinfectants for newborn babies' eyes.[3]

Burns and wound healing make up a multi-billion-dollar industry. One of the foremost treatments is silver, which is used topically as a gel, liquid, spray, bandage, and antimicrobial to enhance wound healing. Because silver destroys bacteria, viruses, and yeast it will help any wound or burn by preventing infection and stimulating stem cells.[133] Wounds heal faster and with less scarring when bacteria, viruses and yeast cannot contaminate the wound. Burn victims report a reduction in pain when silver liquid or gel is applied to the wound. Because silver can be applied in an open wound it can assist in disinfection and help stimulate the healing factors of the immune system. This is true for vaginal infections and internal bleeding in the uterus or cervix as well.

New advances with silver continue to be made in the pursuit of maximum effectiveness and safety. In just the past two or three years, brand new ways of structuring silver molecules into water have been developed that show significantly improved results when compared with earlier silver products. This is an emerging field in terms of public familiarity.

Critical Differentiations: Structured Silver is New

This brings us to a critical point: structured silver is not the same as other silver products. Even other products that contain silver and water are not the same as structured silver.

1000 years ago, people used primitive forms of silver and received mild antimicrobial benefits.

100 years ago, people used primitive colloidal and ionic silver products and received good antimicrobial benefits, but also suffered side effects like Argyria. Argyria is not life-threatening and is rare, but it is an undesirable discoloration of the skin towards a bluish-grey. Argyria can occur with concentrated silvers (very high ppm, such as 50,000 ppm) and impure silver compounds (eg. silver salts) that precipitate within the

body. Argyria cannot happen with new structured silvers, when taken as suggested.

10 years ago, people used more advanced silver solutions and gels and received excellent antimicrobial benefits and vastly improved safety standards.

Today, people have access to structured silver products that even outperform last decade's products. The new silvers are safer and more effective. When compared with last decade's top products at top U.S. laboratories and in clinical usage, today's structured silver shows significantly improved performance against pathogens and reduced healing times as high as 40% faster.

In short, our ability to access silver's benefits has moved from primitive to good over the centuries, with new levels of excellence available now that are even better than last decade's best. Just as computers have developed at a rapid pace, so have silvers. A computer from 25 or 10 years ago was a good tool at the time, but how many people choose an old computer when faced with a design, communication, programming, or entertainment need? 10 years old may be good, but it is no longer the best. As it is with computers, cameras, and smartphones, so it is with silvers.

When choosing your silver products, be mindful of what you seek. You might not be able to see the differences with the naked eye, but they are real and can impact your health.

If you were five or six nanometers tall, the differences between silver products would be as obvious as the differences between a horse and a cow. Yet, since you are likely closer to five or six feet tall, the differences between a pH-balanced (alkaline) structured silver and other substances are invisible without closer inspection.

In short, you do not need to use your grandma's silver. Just as horses and cows are similar yet critically different, old-fashioned silver products and pH-balanced structured silver are similar but critically different from one another.

With clarity on this point, a new health vector emerges. Without clarity, today's new silver products are incorrectly called "snake oil" or worse due to confusion with older technologies.

Unfortunately, many of today's medical experts remain ignorant of the interrelationship between physics, energy, healing, and silver. When questioned about silver, many experts still respond in terms of biochemistry, which is a decades-old approach suitable for decades-old silvers that worked through biochemistry. However, the biochemical paradigm is insufficient for understanding and applying today's silvers, which are built with biophysics in mind.

This is a huge shortcoming of today's medical field. Leading-edge doctors are making use of the latest silver technologies, but many more doctors still think in an obsolete paradigm.

Beyond Just Chemistry

As methods of using silver have advanced over the centuries, the primary focus has been on chemistry. Whether dealing with basic metallurgy or finding ways to access silver within a liquid, the questions have generally centered around "what are the ingredients" and "what size are the particles." These questions led us from using silver coins in our water supplies (the root of today's odd practice of throwing coins into public fountains) to basic colloidal silver products, ionic silver liquids, and even to nanosilver solutions. These advances led humanity from primitive access of silver to a much better form.

However, the progress does not stop with chemistry. Newer forms of silver are also utilizing physics to even further improve our access to silver. In addition to the questions of ingredients and size, leaders in the field are now also asking, "How does biophysics apply?"

For instance, did you know that silver is the best conductor of energy on the entire Periodic Table of the Elements, yet that most of today's silver products do not take advantage of this? Most of today's popular silver products also do not take advantage of recent breakthroughs in magnetics that profoundly affect molecular structure, the characteristics of water, and ultimately the ability of an end product to defeat pathogens.

Summarized, by the year 2013 there were several silver products on the market with excellent chemistry, but very few with equally excellent physics. The difference in performance is clear in lab results and clinical healing times, but many people are not yet accustomed to thinking in terms of biophysics and thus find these performance differences confusing.

If you are new to the term "biophysics," I suggest taking a few minutes to do an online search for the topic. It will prove most illuminating.

Very briefly, biophysics strives to address biological questions while using tools and principles from physics. This includes magnetism, wavelengths (including x-rays and MRI), nanotechnology, and energy. Biophysics is already used in hospitals throughout North America, yet most people are still more accustomed to thinking of health within the biochemistry model that was dominantly explored and taught throughout the 20th century.

What Does Silver Do?

Silver destroys germs (bacteria, viruses, yeast and some parasites). These germs may be living in the pores (causing acne), in the vagina (causing a vaginal infection), in an eye (causing pinkeye), in the digestive tract (causing gas or a serious health problem), in a wound (obstructing healing or causing scarring), around a piercing (causing infection), on the cuticles (causing inflamed hangnails), on the lips (causing cold sores), in the bladder (causing bladder infection), on the toenails (causing odor or unsightly infections), etc.

Regardless of where they are growing, the problem is the same: germs are growing and disrupting your health.[4, 5]

If you can name a spot in or on your body and you can get silver into contact with germs that are growing there, this is where silver can help you. If you keep silver in contact with the germs for six minutes, these germs will no longer be able to cause you health problems.

Simply by killing germs, an amazing list of health problems can be helped or avoided.

Which Germs?

Silver has been shown to be effective with several categories of pathogens (bacteria, viruses and yeast). This includes several hundred pathogens once the various species are all counted. In contrast to conventional antibiotics that typically have a limited spectrum of activity (they only kill about 20 of the 654 bacteria and no viruses nor yeast), this is unexpected and exciting.

Summarized, silver is a broad-spectrum antimicrobial that:

- Destroys pathogenic bacteria
- Inhibits viral replication
- Destroys many fungi, yeasts, and protozoa

· Destroys the malaria parasite

Silver even kills antibiotic-resistant strains of bacteria such as MRSA. Antibiotic resistance is a major problem facing hospitals and homes around the world, as pathogenic bacteria no longer respond to antibiotics such as penicillin, methicillin, vancomycin, and so on. Do an online news search for "MRSA" or "superbugs" and you will see how serious the problem is. Some bacterial infections no longer respond to any drugs, and the problem is getting worse. However, due to the fact that structured silver kills bacteria differently than traditional antibiotics, it kills resistant and non-resistant bacteria alike. This paragraph could easily be expanded into a book of its own, but the simple and relevant fact is this: structured silver eliminates pathogenic bacteria, including drug-resistant strains.

Yet, despite this incredible ability to kill pathogens, structured silver is safe enough to be used at home on a daily basis, does not require a prescription, and is cost-effective.

Alkalinity

Most silver liquids used by the public today are acidic, meaning they have a pH of less than 7.0. The healing process could be improved with an alkaline silver. To do this the water has to be structured in a specific way and stay at a pH above 7.0. After such production, Nelson labs found it to kill more completely than any other silver tested by log 1.4 (1.4 million more bacteria died from the pH-balanced or alkaline silver).

The human body is neutral at a pH of 7.4. When the body is in balance at the average pH of 7.4 the body absorbs what it should and rejects the toxins or poisons and destroys abnormal cells in a preventive and regenerative fashion. When an acid is introduced to the body by eating or drinking it creates a change in metabolism, immunity and circulation. Poisons, toxins and infectious diseases do not survive in an alkaline body solution of pH 7.5 or higher. For this reason it makes sense to have silver be delivered into the body at an alkaline pH. It is true that most all silver solutions are acidic (pH 4.5 - 6.0), and they have performed excellently, but the new alkaline silver works with the body systems even better than the acid silver. By using pH-balanced silver the body can utilize its natural healing mechanisms in cooperation with the antimicrobial silver. In so doing there is a synergistic effect that destroys pathogens more completely in cooperation with the healing processes that excel in alkalinity. The body does not have to convert nor compete with an acid during the prevention and healing mechanisms.

Silver Energy

The energy within silver comes in several forms. It can be electric, magnetic, electromagnetic, chemical, resonant frequency, can steal electrons or fire electrons. It can be acidic or alkaline. These energies can be produced from within the silver and can be dipolar and semiconducting. The energy surrounding silver begins with the atomic structure of silver, where it is missing a single electron in its outer ring. This makes silver continuously hungry to find a single electron. The energy of the silver molecule craves a single electron and will steal it from the easiest source available. When silver moves into close proximity with free-roaming electrons the silver will rapidly bind to the rogue electron. In this way silver is always on patrol surveying the bloodstream for electrons. When silver comes in contact with bacteria, viruses or yeast there will be an attempt by the silver to steal an electron from the pathogen. Since pathogens have simple cell walls made of single electrons, when silver steals an electron it ruptures the pathogens' cell membrane, like puncturing a water balloon. This usually kills the pathogen. The reason that silver doesn't kill healthy cells is because healthy cells have a lipid bilayer. So healthy cells have two layers made from lipids. The fact that there are two separate and distinct layers means that the silver can only steal one electron, and this is not sufficient to rupture or damage the healthy cell walls. In addition, the lipids are fats and silver is usually carried in a water-soluble form that cannot penetrate through the fat bilayers. This is another reason that silver doesn't kill the good probiotic bacteria in the intestines. The genus Lactobacillus is a unique healthy gut bacteria, in that it is the only classification of bacteria that secretes a coating onto its own outer cell wall. The coating is a kind of milk fat that water-soluble silver will not penetrate. This is why the structured silver does not destroy the good bacteria in the gut.

Magnetic energy is being used throughout medicine. It is the gold standard for MRI scanning and helps reduce pain. The magnetic silver energy holds the silver atoms together in molecular crystal structures made of Ag_4O_4, Ag_4O_6, Ag_2O_4 and other antimicrobial structures. The magnetic charge resonates between two phases of silver (silver I and silver III). This makes it a pulse magnet vibrating (resonating) between the two phases of silver, producing antimicrobial and pain-killing abilities.

When the electrical charges that cause the silver to bond to pathogens rather than healthy tissues work together with the magnetic silver energy that sends miniscule pulses of a healthy electromagnetic frequency, it weakens, dissolves and dismantles cellular structures of germs.

This silver energy that destroys pathogens is a resonant frequency. Everything has its own unique frequency and silver vibrates (resonates) at a frequency of approximately 910 terahertz. This is an ultraviolet frequency that destroys pathogens by producing a vibration that weakens, dissolves and dismantles germs (bacteria, viruses, some parasites and yeast). (R. Roy, Anisodesmicity) There are healthy frequencies and destructive frequencies and every cell responds differently to each frequency. The healthy cells with lipid bilayers respond to ultraviolet frequencies in a healthy manner. Silver energy resonates at an antimicrobial ultraviolet frequency. Healthy skin cells respond to ultraviolet energy in a healthy way: they secrete Vitamin D and other healthy immune systemic effects. Pathogens respond to ultraviolet silver energy in a destructive manner, presumably because of the thin single cell walls that are easily ruptured by silver vibration. In this way silver resonates at one frequency but produces healthy results in normal cells and can destroy the cellular structures of pathogens.

Another energy affecting the function of silver is magnetic. Science has demonstrated in many ways that miniscule magnetic energy can have significant impacts on normal cells causing the production and mobilization of stem cells, natural killer cells, lymphocytes and white blood cells. Homeopathic medicine is founded on the principle that miniscule chemical, electric or magnetic charges have long-term health benefits, while great adjustments in any of these energies can cause short-term changes with temporary benefits. An example is antibiotics that have a large effect but can only be supported by the immune and digestive systems for a few weeks or the results are more damaging than the disease. So silver has a miniscule magnetic charge that helps align chemical bonds in the cells, tissues, body systems and even between the atoms influencing molecular structures. When the magnetic charges are coupled with electric charges and are supported by the body in the proper pH, the silver will gather atoms into organized structures called crystalline structures. These structures consist of 2, 4 or 6 silver atoms bonded with water into tetrahedral structures resulting in a multivalent, semiconducting, electromagnetically-charged particle that possesses stronger pathogen-killing abilities. It can also recharge itself for longer more potent killing effects. These structures of 2, 4, or 6 silver atoms gain the ability to repeatedly fire silver electrons, or rupture germ cells by stealing electrons. The silver structure resonates between atomic phases producing a semiconductor so tiny it fits inside a single cell and circulates throughout all of the circulatory system. Imagine a germ killer small enough to fit inside a single red blood cell and resonate at an antimicrobial frequency that travels everywhere blood flows. This means there is electrical energy within the silver structure which causes electrons to continuously circulate around the atomic structure of the silver crystal. The silver structure propels electrons at the speed of light back and forth between the silver I phase and the silver III phase, giving an overall measurement of silver II. When the electrons within the silver structure resonate between the silver atoms at the speed of light there is an active energy being generated within the silver structure. There are significant increases in chemical, electrical, magnetic, electromagnetic energies that are functioning as semiconductors of complex energy. In this way the structured silver possesses sufficient energy to destroy bacteria, viruses, yeast, mold and even some parasites. The structure of the silver is essential to this higher level of antimicrobial activity. The simple forms of silver that are not structured have limited transient and temporary antimicrobial activity. By bonding the silver into structured forms it minimizes Argyria. In other words, when silver is bonded in structured molecular forms the water molecules permanently bond to the silver atoms and will not let the silver separate from the silver structure. This almost eliminates the problem of Argyria because the silver stays with the water molecule and is excreted the same as drinking water. The silver, in structured form, makes a silver solution, while the unstructured forms of silver produce silver suspensions that allow the silver to fall out of solution and as they separate and bind to the body fat they can become permanently bonded to the fats and cause the blue-grey skin color associated with Argyria.

In homeopathic medicine the energy and dilution determine the effectiveness of the solution. Structured Silver has an energy that is homeopathic. This silver energy can be used as medicine in solutions that have been through succussion, and diluted to parts per million that produce medicinal effects that are reproducible.

I performed my Internship in Cardiology at LDS Hospital (University of Utah), where my major professors were Dr. Frank Yanowitz and Nobel Laureate Dr. Jonas Salk. Dr. Salk has been credited with the cure for polio. As I worked with him he taught me how a virus could be diluted in half and again in half and again as many times as it took to leave 1 part per million of the virus in a liquid dilution. This was so diluted that there was hardly any of the virus left in the bottle, but when injected into mice would still cause the polio virus to infect the mice. Dr. Salk showed me how the bottles that were so diluted were randomly stored next to bottles with no virus and the virus would translocate from one bottle that had virus across glass bottles into a different bottle of water with no virus. Yes, it seems impossible that a glass bottle containing water only, could be stored next to the active diluted virus and over a short period of time the water could test positive for the virus but had no virus in it. This example demonstrates an energy that resonates in the virus that can electromagnetically leave the active virus and enter the water bottle. This is how we end up with a vaccine that transfers the energy of the virus without infecting the person receiving the vaccination. Then over time the immune system mounts an immune response that renders immunity against the poliovirus. As you can see silver can deliver an energy that can destroy pathogens, stimulate the immune system and resonate at a frequency that destroys pathogens and promotes healthy stem cells and lymphocytes at the same time. This is the magic of silver energy.

In addition, the silver energy functions better when the human body is kept alkaline (pH 7.2-7.5). In this way the body will create an environment that is unfriendly for pathogens and the silver can perform its antimicrobial actions more efficiently. Another assist to silver energy is antioxidants. By regularly consuming natural antioxidants the body will be able to reduce inflammation and quickly excrete the dead pathogens that were killed by the silver energies. This is important because it significantly reduces the symptoms associated with die-off of pathogens. The antioxidants are the perfect partner for silver energy because the silver kills and the antioxidants clear out the die-off and reduce the inflammation of the disease state, which significantly reduces the cause of the symptoms associated with the healing process. In summary, there are numerous silver energies that destroy bacteria, viruses, yeast, mold and some parasites while selectively sparing the healthy cells, and this process can be improved when the body is in an alkaline (not acidic) state. The symptoms, inflammation and healing times are improved when antioxidants are taken every four hours. To destroy the cause of many disease states and promote prevention, wisdom suggests an alkaline body, with regular supplements of silver and antioxidants.

Characteristics of Silver Energy:

- Redox reaction (silver I to silver III)
- Electric
- Magnetic (pulse magnetic)
- Electromagnetic
- Resonant frequency
- Alkaline over acid
- Ultraviolet antimicrobial resonant frequency
- Steals electrons from pathogens
- Fires electrons into pathogens, fracturing the cell wall
- As a semi-conductor, produces singlet oxygen that kills complex diseases
- Silver energy is water-soluble and does not penetrate healthy bacteria or cells
- Acidic silver is almost as good as structured alkaline (pH-balanced) silver energy but acidic silver triggers immune responses that promote autoimmunity and

can cause chemical burns as an acid
- Alkaline silver works with the immune system as it destroys pathogens

All silver does not have the same energies.

Ionic Silver: consists of chemical energy that is mostly electric and can be measured by its charge. The problem is that it bonds to the fats and is the primary cause of Argyria.

Colloidal Silver: consists of electric currents driving silver ions into water. Some colloids are nothing more than tiny particles of silver dusting the water that contains them. If the wrong electrical current is used to manufacture the colloid the silver will fall out of solution and can become predominantly ionic.

Structured Silver: is an advanced second-generation colloidal silver that is magnetically and electrically structured, producing atomic bonding of water and silver in a way that forms crystalline structures of silver and water. The structured silver bonds permanently to the water so it forms a solution of silver hydrosol, which has alkaline properties. The magnetic and electric frequencies used during manufacturing are combined with a structured water that results in alkaline, magnetic, electric silver in a structured form. It is significantly more effective at destroying pathogens than the colloids and ionics of the past. The reason is that the structured silver holds an ultraviolet antimicrobial frequency, capable of working with the immune system because it is alkaline.

Structured Silver Water: What a Structure Means

Structured silver water contains a specialized natural and purified water that contains nanoparticles of silver permanently distributed into the water at the molecular level. This structured silver water is chemically different than ionic or colloidal forms of silver because the water that makes up 99.9% of the silver solution has been electrically, magnetically, mechanically and physically activated using scientific methods that result in a unique water structure that permanently holds the pure silver in a molecular structure that has been shown to have antimicrobial effects inside or outside the body. This unique type of structured, alkaline, silver water is identified in crystalline molecular structures consisting of similar atoms with movable crystal structures.

For example, silver colloid allows the silver to fall out of its bond with water and the Ag H2O becomes Ag – H-O-H. This is why colloidal and ionic silver cause Argyria (silver staining of the skin)—the silver falls out of solution with the water and the renegade silver finds fats to bond with. The colloidal and ionic forms of silver separate from the water, possibly causing problems under the skin.

The new structured alkaline silver water prevents this from happening because the silver is permanently (magnetically, electrically and chemically) bonded to the purified structured water. This results in tetrahedral-shaped water molecules called crystals or crystalline structures. The tetrahedral-shaped molecules keep 4 water molecules bonded to 2, 4, or 6 silver (Ag) atoms, permanently bonding water, silver, hydrogen and oxygen atoms into structured silver molecules (Ag4O2, Ag4O4, Ag4O6). The fluid dynamic of this structured silver water allow some atoms from the Ag4O6 to translocate and become Ag4O4 or Ag4O2. This allows the structure of the water to hold the silver in a crystal shape that has thousands of times more antimicrobial effects than just silver in an ionic or colloidal shape.

It is much safer because it keeps the silver in the water, where it will be excreted from the body quickly. The structure of the water is held together by electric, magnetic and chemical bonds, creating a situation for alternative energies to be imprinted upon the crystalline structure in cooperation with the silver. Electric, magnetic and light waves can be imprinted into the chemical atoms or used to hold the bonds together between the atoms, thus improving the molecular bond angles, strength or shapes. This changes the crystalline shapes of the water and gives it a structure with purpose. The frequency of the bond, the shape of the water crystal and the magnetic strength of the atomic bonds produce a unique structure and specific purpose to the structured silver water.

The structured silver water has scientifically proven antimicrobial effects that are improved when it is placed in an alkaline solution. The combination of alkalinity and structured water produce a frequency that is easily absorbed into the body because of its optimal alkaline balance (7.5 pH). This produces a structured silver water that tests far better than any other silver for its ability to destroy bacteria, viruses and yeast. Since these are the causes of most all diseases, it provides the body with the very best all-natural solution to destroy the most disease-causing pathogens, and to work in cooperation with the chemical structure of all body systems at pH 7.5.

Magnetism

Magnetic fields are significant to the human body and have been proven to improve healing, reduce pain and are used to treat, diagnose and identify different types of cells. The magnetic resonance imager (MRI) scans the body and dissects the individual cell types using magnetic fields. It is one of the fastest growing specialties in traditional medicine.

Magnetic fields of different frequencies have been shown to influence the body in dramatic clinical ways, such as mental illness, pain reduction, sleep and mood. This technology can complement and magnify the positive effects of structured silver. By choosing the proper magnetic frequency and imprinting the water and silver atoms, the strength of bonds and the angles can change the shape of the crystalline structure within the silver and water. This can produce electron donors and acceptors that produce quantum mechanical changes with the structured silver water.

During an increase in the energy or the structured silver solution an excited molecular structure progresses to create an extended outer orbital, which resonates at a frequency of higher energy. As the energy in the outer orbital is released, an electron is fired into the pathogen, killing it and releasing a subatomic high-energy particle.

This stealing of electrons from the disease-causing pathogens and firing into them is only accomplished by structured silver water. Colloidal and ionic silvers can steal one electron from a pathogen and then become neutral, while the structured silver water can continuously steal electrons from the pathogens and then fire back at high energy and resonate at an antimicrobial frequency; a magnetic signature can also be imprinted on the subatomic bonds, giving them magnetic influence at the cellular level. These signatures can influence pain, strength, balance, and do so because the mitochondria (powerhouse of the cell) have improved function.

This improved function has been shown to have improvements on health, wellness, energy levels and promote cellular energies that have great purposes for healing.

Electrical Energy

Electrical energy can be imprinted upon the structured silver water, giving it a tremendous output of electrical energy that can benefit the healing process. Healing sciences have demonstrated that miniscule electrical currents passing through the human body have significant healing activity. The body is electrical and conducts electrical energy through the fluids in the body as long as there is a substantial amount of minerals dissolved in the body fluids. Since the body is predominantly water with iron and salts dissolved into the blood, a miniscule electrical current can be conducted through the entire body.

Electromagnetic Energy

When the electric and magnetic are tuned to a healing frequency that the body recognizes, every cell in the body can have the influence of that healing frequency. Results include stronger muscle contractions, more coordinated neuromuscular function that can result in better balance, and healing at the cellular level. There are many frequencies that have been identified as having clinical benefits to the human body, such as improved healing, breathing, balance, mental focus, memory enhancement, cell regeneration, skin and wound healing and mitochondrial energy production. Some physics books even identify frequencies that destroy cancer cells, infectious diseases, or viral infections, thus eliminating the cause of the disease.

When the chemical energy is optimal, the electrical energy promotes healing, and the magnetic energy is beneficial to the body and is conducted throughout the human body by nanoparticles of silver that have antibacterial, antiviral and antifungal properties, there you will find structured silver water in an alkaline balance. And the laboratories report this is the finest full-spectrum antimicrobial when compared to other forms of silver.

Industrial Hygiene During Manufacturing Why Manufacturing Has To Be In A Clean Room

The production of structured silver must be manufactured under clean-room conditions utilizing good manufacturing procedures (GMP). This is significant because most silver manufactures don't realize that when the atoms of oxygen, silver and hydrogen are under the influence of electric, magnetic and chemical energies that any substance in the air, water or production facility could donate contaminants into the silver liquid.

Structured silver uses a unique manufacturing instrument that begins with pure water constructed using steam and oxygen. In this way the hydrogen and oxygen can be precisely formulated into a structured pure water that is measured to have zero total dissolved solids (TDS). This is pure water that is ready to have electric, magnetic and chemical imprints placed with the bonding of the silver. If you do not have a perfectly clean room, you will be drawing atoms from the air, tubes, container, etc. that will pollute the water and coat the silver.

This coating on the surface of the silver interferes with the purity of the silver in the water, thus reducing the effectiveness of the silver to bind with pathogens, thus impeding the effectiveness of the silver for healing purposes. Most silvers have been shown to have a protein coat or are called silver proteins because they are mostly protein. All of these protein coats are direct evidence of polluted and contaminated silver.

If the silver is manufactured in a contaminated room then it produces an inferior product. Structured silver water is produced under clean-room conditions and pure ingredients are used under precise energies to obtain a silver molecule that forms a plasma-like silver without a protein coat to interfere with the effectiveness and killing ability of silver.

Antioxidants and Silver

Silver destroys bacteria, viruses, yeast and some parasites using all-natural ingredients. This remarkable healing effect cannot be achieved by any prescription medication. The killing of the pathogens is essential to healing wounds, controlling infectious diseases and preventing viral, bacterial and fungal diseases. The healing process can be accelerated when there are sufficient antioxidants circulating in the body simultaneously.

Antioxidants neutralize the free-radical damage caused by these pathogens and accelerate the excretion of the dead and dying germs out of the body. This reduces the time it takes to heal. It also reduces the swelling associated with the disease and improves the healing inside or topically. When antioxidants are taken every 5 hours the healing process is significant improved. The antioxidants' ability to heal is improved in addition to the healing activity of the silver liquid and gel.

Ideal healing synergism develops when silver liquid destroys pathogens at the same time high potency antioxidants reduce inflammation and enhance excretion of the dead and dying germs.

Antioxidants enter the individual cells and transport nutrients with them as co-factors. Antioxidants can actively transport the silver into the cell where the cause of disease may be sequestered. Once the silver destroys the pathogen, antioxidants have the ability to reduce the swelling associated with the killing of pathogens. By reducing the swelling and inflammation the body will heal faster and with less permanent scarring.

The antioxidants neutralize any metabolites that may be formed during the killing or excretion process. This is especially significant in the intestines and bloodstream where free radicals are being transported out of the body and some may not quite be dead yet. The damage from this cleansing crisis produces free radicals that cause inflammation in arteries and intestines. The antioxidants can minimize this healing and cleansing crisis and at the same time enhance access to the germs hiding within cells.

Silver Will Not Do...

As a skeptic, you may be thinking that structured silver sounds too good to be true. After all, how can one substance do so much? It may sound like a scam—snake oil, magic tomato juice, mythic elixir, or some other dreamy idea that doesn't actually work in the real world.

Thus, it is likely helpful to list some of the things that structured silver will NOT do. After all, it does not do everything, nor is it a cure-all. Based on the type of questions that newcomers typically ask, it is important to clarify this point to keep expectations in check.

Structured silver kills many germs. Since germs cause a wide range of health problems and complications, structured silver is helpful in many situations. But if a health condition does not have some connections to germs, then there is a fair chance that silver will not directly help with it.

For instance, here is a brief list of things that structured silver does NOT do. The remainder of the book will discuss the many things that structured silver CAN do, but first let's quash the notion that it fixes everything.

Structured silver...

- · Will not pull fats out of the arteries
- · Will not cure diabetes, although it can benefit most of the secondary symptoms

caused by diabetes
- Will not destroy all parasites; it will only destroy some parasites
- Will not cure cancer, but it can kill a major cause of it at the cellular level
- Will not cure mental illness unless the cause of the disease is bacterial, fungal or viral
- Will combat dental infections, but it will not regrow teeth
- Will not help fish
- Will not destroy what it does not come into close proximity with
- Does not totally kill until the structured silver water or gel stays in contact with the pathogen for 6 minutes
- Will not improve athletic performance
- Will not dissolve through the skin because it is not fat-soluble
- Will not compensate for a lack of exercise
- Will not compensate for a terrible diet or poor lifestyle
- Will not replace the need for trusted doctors, hospitals and other health care professionals
- etc.

Please be aware that federal regulations limit dietary supplements to oral administration even if structure function claims may be specific to certain body parts.

This list could go on and on, but the point is clear: silver helps with many health concerns, but it is just one piece of the larger puzzle called "good health."

As you read further into this book and you see dozens or hundreds of applications for structured silver, please remain cognizant of two important facts:

1. The list of applications is long, but it is not thousands or millions of items long. The list is long, but not infinite.

2. The list of applications is limited, yes, but it is not short either. It is not limited to just two or three items. The remarkable fact is that structured silver can actually help with an outrageously long list of health problems, including several of humanity's most expensive, debilitating and lethal conditions.

In sum, structured silver is NOT a cure-all. It does not do everything. Still, it may be the closest thing to a panacea that anyone has discovered in a very long time.

On the topic of what structured silver will not do, here are a few additional items:

- Will not hurt antibiotics (it can enhance some antibiotic function)

- Will not kill all the probiotic (good) bacteria in the gut because it cannot pass through the milk fat coating of the Lactobacillus
- Will not kill living normal tissues
- Will not hurt dogs, cats, horses and other mammals
- Will not be covered by insurance

Travel Kit

Travel is supposed to be a pleasant experience, whether traveling for education, work, or personal enjoyment. The last thing anyone wants while traveling is a day spent in the washroom or worse. Yet, all too often, that is exactly what happens to people. What a waste!

With structured silver, you now have the ability to dramatically reduce the risk of illness while away from home.

You can easily be exposed to the most dangerous pathogens when traveling, creating considerable personal risk. This is because you have likely not been exposed to these pathogens before and you have not had a chance to build immunity. Compounding the problem, you may be traveling in a place where you do not want to be placed in the care of poor medical treatment where they may not speak your language.

Silver should be taken for routine uses while traveling, like shaving, after sun tan lotion, sun burn, dry skin, fever blisters, rash, pain, hand sanitizer, vaginal wellness and protection, prevention in the airplane, body odor, yeast infections or petential proximity to foreign pathogens.

Silver liquid and gel should be taken on trips for accidental or infectious reasons, like cuts, colds, flu, blisters, food poisoning, urinary tract infection, pneumonia, wounds, sex, and eyes, ears, nose and throat protection.

- Silver liquid less than 4 oz. bottles for air travel, more for drinking, washing wounds, eyes, ears, nose and throat. Or, place larger bottles in your checked luggage
- Silver gel 2-4 oz. for feet, condoms, vagina, hands and skin.

If it were me, I would swallow the liquid silver two teaspoons twice a day for prevention. If I was sleep-deprived, under stress or exposed to potential disease, I would double the dose to four teaspoons twice a day. In the event I contracted food poisoning, I would take one ounce once every hour for four hours and do that each day for three days. Other options are listed in the "Silver Uses" section of this book.

If you are traveling with others, it is good to discuss silver supplies before leaving home. If someone in your family or travel group becomes infected, do you have enough silver packed to provide assistance? If traveling with family, why not do the math beforehand and potentially save yourselves a lot of trouble?

Medical Missions and Travel Medicine with Dr. Bryan Frank

Some of the most meaningful International travel I have taken has come in the form of humanitarian trips where silver's benefits were brought to people in impoverished conditions. I have witnessed many dramatic recoveries from infectious conditions of all types.

To address the topics of travel and humanitarian medical efforts, I have invited Dr. Bryan Frank, M.D., to share his experiences with silver. Dr. Frank has been performing medical missions on five continents for several decades and I can think of no one more qualified to address this topic—a topic with such dramatic potential to improve conditions for the world's impoverished.

Silver as a Preferred Tool in International Medical Missions and Travel Medicine By Bryan L. Frank, M.D.

Introduction

Aquasols of the last decade, and now the even more effective structured alkalinized silver, have presented in both basic research and clinical experience as remarkable therapeutics in many diverse clinical situations. Silver demonstrates antibacterial, antiviral and antifungal effects for virtually every surface and tissue of the body. Silver is both highly effective clinically and is without toxicity. These properties make silver a preferred therapeutic for treating patients, healthcare volunteers and team members in international missions and humanitarian efforts.

International mission efforts often serve those with little or no access to healthcare, especially from conventional medicine. Tribal or traditional remedies may often be practiced, some of which are, in fact, very beneficial. Silver has similarly been a traditional healing therapeutic for millennia worldwide. With silver, patients may realize profound benefits and avoid the hazards of inferior colloidal and ionic silver preparations. Some traditional cultures (especially in India) have used silver foil as a dietary product for supporting gut health, yet some of the foil is of poor quality and it is not uncommon to see those with Argyria—darkening of the skin in a blue-gray coloration—in those using the inferior silver products.

This chapter is intended to inform of the benefits that may be realized in using silver in international mission and humanitarian projects. We have found silver to be highly effective, without toxicity and therefore extremely safe, and at a good value when compared to expensive pharmaceuticals that are commonly used on these mission projects.

An Integrative Travel and Mission Physician

This author is a medical missionary with over thirty years of experience in a U.S.-based private practice of anesthesiology, pain medicine, integrative anti-aging medicine and medical acupuncture, as well as in extensive travel medicine and medical missions. In his private medical practice, Dr. Frank is President of Re-Genesis Health: New Beginnings in Health and Wellness and is Medical Director of Full Circle Health Clinic in Edmond, OK, working alongside a Naturopathic Physician and Chiropractor, as well as with therapists for massage therapy, colon hydrotherapy, energetic balancing, detox foot therapy and IV infusions for autoimmune conditions, Parkinson's, Fibromyalgia/Chronic Fatigue Syndrome, Hepatitis C, Lyme Disease, cancer and more. He is one of a few physicians in the U.S. to include IV Laser Blood Therapy through his association with the developers in Germany.

As President of Global Mission Partners, Inc. (GMP), a 501(c)(3) nonprofit charitable corporation that serves the poor in developing parts of Asia, Africa, South America and North America, he has used silver for maintaining health and/ or treating a wide variety of medical conditions around the world. He has traveled to more than 55 countries and his teams with GMP currently serve Nepal, India, Kenya, Ecuador and Mexico. He has previously served also in Russia, Haiti, the Dominican Republic, Costa Rica, Appalachia and Native American reservations.

Some of our most exciting work with silver has been for the treatment of malaria in western Kenya. In the tiny village of Kano, near Kisumu on the northeastern shores of Lake Victoria, children and adults have been treated with silver for malaria and are involved in a current clinical research project. To date, most patients have been clinically responsive and returned to work or school within 24-48 hours and their blood tests for plasmodium have reverted to negative within 5-10 days. (More to be discussed on this later in this chapter.)

GMP receives applications for participation in its projects from physicians, dentists, nurses, therapists and non-medical general helper volunteers, as well as students and pastors. GMP also receives financial donations and is supported with silver for its projects by Muvezi Health Projects Society for caring for those with little or no access to healthcare around the globe.

Dr. Frank has extensive travel and trekking experience, treating team members while on treks in the Himalayas, Mont Blanc or Machu Picchu, or while in bustling cities or tiny oxcart villages of Asia, Africa and Latin America. He has authored the Chapter on Pain Management in Wilderness and Travel Medicine in the renowned and definitive text, Wilderness Medicine, 4th and 5th Editions, edited by the highly acclaimed Stanford Emergency Physician, Dr. Paul Auerbach.

As President of Acupuncture Medical Arts, LLC, Dr. Frank has written numerous articles on Medical Acupuncture, Prolotherapy, Neural Therapy, and other related techniques and has published reference charts, The Atlas of Auricular Therapy and Auricular Medicine and the appraised text, Auricular Medicine and Auricular Therapy: A Practical Approach.

Dr. Frank has led medical delegations to Russia, China and Japan for exchanging research and clinical expertise in medical acupuncture. He has lectured across North America and internationally to medical congresses, symposia and seminars to many thousands of physicians and other healthcare workers in Europe, Asia, Oceana and North and South America. He served as President of the American Academy of Medical Acupuncture/AAMA (1999-2001), President of the International Council of Medical Acupuncture and Related Techniques/ICMART (2004-2006) and also as Vice-President of ICMART (2002-2004 and 2010-2012).

Dr. Frank is an ordained and licensed pastor, serving as Global Missions Pastor and Healing House Pastor for Citychurch in Oklahoma City, OK. Over the last 30 years, he has led hundreds of volunteers to serve thousands of needy people in over 100 missions for healthcare, construction, street children and orphanage, water well, community development, women's skills development, education, micro-loan finance, as well as preaching, teaching and Christian discipleship.

The Role of Silver in Missionary or Travel Medicine

One role of silver that may be neglected as teams organize and prepare for mission projects is that of preventing disease and maintaining good health in the participants prior to, throughout and following the mission project. With this consideration, the author encourages all team members to begin taking 1-2 tablespoons of silver twice daily in the week prior to the project, continuing throughout and then following the project for at least one to two weeks. This is important, as some organisms may be latent and not expressing clinical illness until some days after return from a mission project.

Clearly, silver has great applications for treating patients on the mission field as well. GMP has experience using silver on malaria in Kenya, upper and lower respiratory infections in Ecuador, skin lesions in India and more. The widely effective use of silver for infections from bacteria, virus and fungus are seen to be effective on any surface and any tissue. We have used SILVER orally, topically as liquid or gel on skin, vagina or rectum, inhaled or sprayed into the nose or mouth and dropped in the eyes and ears. Silver is well received and is without taste and without pain or irritation on any bodily surface or tissue.

It is not uncommon, especially in small health camps in primitive oxcart villages, to be without sophisticated bio-diagnostic tools and instruments. As such, at times a definitive diagnosis is difficult, and a clinical diagnosis or differential is only available. Because silver has a broad spectrum of clinical efficacy, we feel confident in using it when we are unable to finalize a diagnosis.

A further advantage or benefit is the relative cost of silver compared to conventional pharmaceuticals. Discounts for case purchases also further good stewardship of funds through the use of silver. Additionally, through the generosity of Muvezi Health Projects Society, donations of silver are being made available to humanitarian projects around the globe.

Prior studies also show silver aquasols to be effective and safe when used in conjunction with other pharmaceuticals. Further, with the absence of toxicity, no side effects are to be expected. This is remarkable, especially when considering the wide range of side effects experienced with pharmaceuticals, some of which are mild, but others quite serious, even lethal. Hippocrates' charge to "first, do no harm" may be followed with ease with silver and give comfort to the physician caring for those with little resources to manage serious side effects.

Silver has also changed Global Mission Partners' practice of vaccination usage among staff and team. In the past, anti-malarial medications or vaccines for yellow fever, typhoid, hepatitis and others would have been typically used. As we now always travel with silver, our position is to not take the other vaccines and medications as preventatives. It is imperative to take all reasonable precautions to prevent contracting infectious diseases, including but not limited to thorough hand washing, covering of nose and mouth with coughs and sneezing, thorough washing of utensils and dishes, use of mosquito netting where indicated, use of mosquito repellents (natural, non-toxic), et cetera.

A Challenge to International Mission and Humanitarian Projects

Given the volumes of science, our years of safe experience with silver, the governmental recognitions, the broad spectrum of indications for its use and the reasonable cost value, I strongly encourage international mission agencies and humanitarian projects to seriously consider using silver on a regular basis. This recommendation includes not only the use in field settings or village health camps, but also for staff and personnel in the international placements with regular, daily use of silver for preventive measures. The daily small use may be increased from 1-2 teaspoons twice daily to 1-2 tablespoons twice daily or more, as indicated. In addition, use of silver gel, drops or sprays may be indicated, depending on site and clinical presentation of the infection.

Silver is not only useful in mission projects that are overtly medical in nature. Any international project should seriously consider the benefits of regular, daily silver use as a preventative health practice as well as prompt increase if and when an indicated health problem arises. Simply stated, silver is safe, effective and cost-conscious. Management of all companies having personnel or other stakeholders' personnel in areas known to have infectious disease should make this silver available. It is not only morally correct but is also financially wise.

Stories from the Mission Field

Kenya: In the tiny village of Kano, near Kisumu on the shores of Lake Victoria, GMP teams have worked with Maisha International, which serves in health camps, water wells, latrines, meals for orphans and widows with AIDS, education and school support and ministry. As we arrived for another mission in July, 2010, and in following projects in 2011 and 2012, numerous children and adults in the village had illness consistent with malaria. Malaria is endemic to the region and while diagnosis of the plasmodium in the blood and medications are available, many go without diagnosis and treatment due to extreme poverty. In this setting, GMP took silver donated by Muvezi Health Projects Society to treat these patients. Diagnosis was made and patients were then treated with 1 tablespoon (15 ml) of structured silver twice daily. We encouraged them to hold the liquid in their mouth for a minute prior to swallowing for absorption to begin across the mucous membranes rapidly.

In our initial trail of approximately 30 patients over the week, all patients became clinically well and were able to return to school or work within 24-48 hours. We were surprised that this was the case even in those patients that appeared clinically worse than others. Repeat blood studies were obtained and found to be reverted to normal in 5 days for most, and 10 days for others. Due to extreme poverty, donations are necessary to provide for the testing as the people live very pragmatically and when they are once well, they are unable to consider the cost of the test in light of needing their next meal, perhaps the only one for the day or for several days. Further testing and treatment is ongoing and it is hoped that a clinical pilot study may be published in the next year from these results in Kenya.

Ecuador: Deep in the jungles of southeastern Ecuador, el Oriente is a land that is home to the Shuar tribal peoples. While Ecuador has roughly 10% of its population from European extraction, about 90% are indigenous peoples of approximately 27 different tribes across the nation. Some of these are high mountain peoples, such as the Quichua of the Andes; others are Amazonian. Unfortunately, the economic reality is inverted, as roughly 90% of the wealth of the nation is in the hands of the minority and only 10% of the wealth is in the hands of the majority indigenous peoples. Such a situation leads to extreme poverty, subsistence living and farming, and lack of basic needs, including medical needs.

The Shuar of el Oriente were head-hunters until a generation ago. Now, many live in government-protected reservations, much as is seen with many Native American tribal peoples. Yet, without casino gaming, oil and gas and other economic resources as are now going to American Native peoples, this is not the case in Ecuador.

GMP has served in Ecuador for 14 years, first high in the Andes at elevations of 9,000 to 12,000 feet, home of the beautiful Quichua peoples. For the last three years, GMP now serves the Shuar in the cool, dry and gorgeous jungles. In our project in June 2010, a small boy came to the clinic with a laceration to the foot. While this may be a simple problem for many in North America, lack of health education, even including basic washing and asepsis, is often unknown. His infection demonstrated a nasty wound with the redness of cellulitis around the laceration. Thorough cleaning of the wound was made and silver gel, donated to GMP by Muvezi Health Projects Society, was applied. This was to be reapplied 2-3 times per day, in addition to one tablespoon of liquid silver orally twice daily. The boy experienced clearing of the wound much more rapidly than expected, even from the best of conventional topical antibiotic care.

In general, other applications of silver in Ecuador have included not only topical wound infections, but also eye, ear and nasal purulent infections. The solution is not painful and has been highly effective when used in place of optic or otic antibiotic solutions, such as ciprofloxacin or gentamycin drops.

Nepal: The mysterious Kathmandu sits on a high plain, approximately 4,200 feet above sea level, surrounded by a ring of hills at 8,000 to 12,000 feet high. On a clear day, free from the usual pollution, the Himalayas show their snowy splendor: reaching 18,000 to 29,035 feet, the southern slopes of Mt. Everest, or Sagarmatha to the Nepali, Mother Goddess of the Universe.

GMP has served in over 22 missions to Nepal in the last 15 years. On a project to Nepal in March 2010, a small girl presented with matting and drainage from her eyes. These eye infections are highly contagious even in the U.S., and can spread to all in a family living in small village homes rapidly.

Using a small plastic dropper, silver was dropped into both eyes, 2-3 drops each, 2-3 times per day. As with external ear infections, we have seen the silver drops remedy these infections, typically within 24 hours. Further, the drops do not sting the eyes or the ears and thus they are well tolerated and received.

We have also had patients who do well clinically in Nepal with silver for vaginal and urinary complaints, using the solution both orally and topically, (topical gel for vaginal inflammation or infections). Additionally, our team reports recent successes with silver gel for psoriasis that was resistant to conventional care.

Beyond these common conditions, we have used silver gel with some leprosy patients for their very serious wounds which develop due to sensory and motor nerve defects which accompany this horrible disease. Silver used topically as the gel or as the solution soaking a gauze on the lesion, as well as oral silver, has demonstrated tissue wound healing that often is better than that seen with conventional antibiotic and skin wound care.

Conclusions

Silver solution and gel has proven to be a very valuable therapeutic for both the mission health camps and for the health of the team as it travels. Its wide range of antibacterial, antiviral and antifungal properties make it useful for treating many clinical infections. As it is painless and can be used orally as well as on any body surface or in any body opening, there is wide acceptance for use by patients.

Organizational leaders should seriously consider the use of silver as the first line of defense for their teams and for their patients. In our situation, we have avoided the use of various immunizations and antibiotics and obviously their potential side effects due to the success of silver in treating the various infectious conditions. Included in this is its use for malaria. While we cannot advise anyone to avoid immunizations or antibiotics, and each person should seek the advice of a knowledgeable health care provider, our experience has led us to be confident in this practice whereby we use silver in place of most immunizations and antibiotics. At times, if the silver has not satisfactorily resolved a clinical problem quickly, it may be used in conjunction with other pharmaceuticals with no conflict or harm. As this is an emerging technology that is not yet widely known, I encourage all organizational leaders to share the information about structured silver and its many uses so that their volunteers may be fully informed as to options for their own health as well as that of those they will treat on mission projects.

Silver and the Environment

It has been suggested by outside media groups that silver could pose a threat to the drinking water and environment. Silver poses absolutely no threat to our drinking water, according to numerous sources. There are no health risks, because it (silver) never turns up in any water treatment centers and because it is not being detected in any amount, even at levels as low as one part per billion. It poses no threat.

There are numerous substances found in our water supply and environment which have been listed as potential problems, and silver is not one of them. The water quality experts are watching for trace amounts of antibiotics, anticonvulsants, mood stabilizers, toxins and sex hormones. Ken Bousfield (Department of Environmental Quality) says, "Depending on the pharmaceuticals involved, it would involve perhaps taking an Olympic swimming pool volume of water day in and day out for a period of years before you'd receive a health effect."[6] And silver would take at least ten times more water to an impossible amount to present a potential problem. Potential water toxins are evaluated by their potential for toxicity and the AWWA Research Foundation has identified the 16 most toxic substances in the ground water, and drinking water and silver is not one of them, nor does it appear on any unsafe list since it isn't being found in any detectable amount.

The researchers quantify these substances by a term called drinking water equivalent levels (DWEL). Some of the substances that appear in highest concentrations in our water include Diazepam, Naproxen and Atenolol. Dr. Snyder reports that it would take drinking 110,000 gallons of treated water for thirty years before a person would have a one in a million chance of developing a medical risk[7]. And silver is substantially safer than these treatments by a factor of at least ten times, because ten times less people consume or use it.

Structured alkaline silver is produced in extremely low parts per million (5-40 ppm) and has never even been identified as a potential for problem in the water treatment plants or in the environment. This is significant because the EPA has a rating for toxic spills. This identifies the amount of a compound that would cause a toxic event. For instance, Clorox would qualify as a toxic event if 3 gallons were spilled. In contrast, The EPA would require a spill of 12.5 million gallons of silver in order to be classified as a toxic event.[8] This would require spilling the entire contents of 12.5 oil tankers at one time in one place without any other water to dilute it. There is no consumer or combination of consumers that store this much silver anywhere in the country.

An average water treatment plant treats about 30 to 70 million gallons of water a day and it would take a spill of about 7 tankers full of a structured alkaline silver liquid directly into the treatment water to bring the concentration to 1 part per million. This is still a very safe level for fish, and an impossible event to happen anywhere in the world.

When you look at the source of these suggestions for regulating silver, you will find that many of the proponents of the complaints come from pesticide companies that stand to lose a significant amount of business due to the fact that silver has become certified as a pesticide without harmful side effects to humans. The real threat is to the American people that are being exposed to hazardous pesticides proven to cause cancers, nerve damage, immune disorders and can be fatal to animals and humans.

It is truly criminal to allow the misrepresented facts to continue the support of hazardous pesticide use while there is a safe alternative in silver. When you realize that our ground water comes from the snow that melts on the mountains and is filtered through the vast amount of minerals in our soils, you understand that silver is a major participant in the filtering of our water and it has never appeared in measurable amounts nor is it dangerous. These groups want to promote the use of highly toxic pesticides instead of the harmless silver, and they are demanding regulation of a substance (silver) that is already being certified and safely regulated. It is clearly a case of politics over proof.

The Safe and Non-Toxic Nature of Structured Silver

Structured silver is remarkably safe. It can be used internally or in any orifice of the body—eyes, ears, nose, mouth, rectum, or vagina.

If taken internally, it selectively kills pathogenic bacteria while leaving healthy bacteria ("probiotics") unharmed. This selection happens similar to the way probiotics are able survive within the harsh environment of the stomach and digestive tract. Probiotics have a double layer of fatty protection on their outer edge, whereas pathogenic bacteria do not. This fatty layer protects probiotics from stomach acid, allowing them to grow and contribute to digestion. In the same way, this lipid bi-ayer protects probiotics from the water-based silver product's antibacterial action.

According to the Merck Manual of Diagnosis and Therapy, silver is not considered to be a heavy metal and it does not accumulate in the brain.[9] In fact, it is the only metal that is not considered to be a heavy metal because it does not produce heavy metal poisoning.[10]

According to the IRIS report, silver is non-toxic at 5000mg/kg of body weight and 90-99% of ingested silver leaves the body within 24 hours.[11]

Additionally, silver is already being used in hospitals, space shuttles, washing machines, water filters, and many other settings for its ability to control unwanted microbes. Yet, it is so safe and non-toxic that it would take a spill of over 12 million gallons of 10 ppm silver before the EPA would consider it a reportable spill. (12) In contrast, less one millionth of that amount of spilled bleach requires an EPA report!

Hundreds of scientific studies have been reported to document the benefits and safe use of silver in animals and humans.[13-41] Results of this scientific review demonstrate the safety of structured silver.

Results from safety and toxicology studies demonstrate credible and unanimous safety evidence from experimental testing performed in humans, animals, laboratories, hospitals, medical clinics, in vitro, injected, ingested, cytotoxicity and overdosed sources. Results from all these studies report safe, beneficial and non-toxic data in structured silver as compared to the salt and ionic forms of silver which can accumulate under the skin and cause the discoloration called Argyria.

The only adverse event known, from the medicinal use of silver, is Argyria. EPA reports have determined that administering one gram total elemental silver over a 2-year period presents no risk for developing Argyria.[42] Approximately 99% of all Argyria reports occur in patients that manufactured their own colloidal ionic (salt form) of silver. According to a report from the EPA Registration Eligibility Document (RED), "the Office of Water classified silver as a Group D carcinogen (one that is not classifiable as to carcinogenicity in humans) in 1988." The EPA established an oral Reference Dose (RfD), or daily intake limit, of 0.005 mg/kg/day for silver in 1991.[43] This equates to an equivalent safe daily dose of 1 oz of 10 ppm structured silver.

The conclusion of this review is that the structured alkaline silver liquid technology is safe and non-toxic to healthy human cells, humans, animals, and meets safety standards.

Structured silver fulfills the definition of being non-toxic, in that it passes through the body unchanged, this means it does not produce any harmful metabolites. Marino (Chem. Bioil. Interactions, 1974), and Berger (Antimicrobial Agents, 1976), confirmed that the effective dosage level of pure silver is safe for mammalian tissues. The CRC Handbook to Chemistry and Physics (sec. 15, pg. 8) states: "While silver is not considered to be toxic, most of its salts are poisonous." This is why structured, pH-balanced silver containing only elemental silver and pure structured water is virtually devoid of toxicity.

Nanoparticles

The definition of a nanoparticle is that it must be a tiny .05 nanometers in size.

This means that only the smallest of particles can be placed under the label of nanoparticle. Some media groups suggest that a nanoparticle of a specific size (.001 nm) can be dangerous by collecting and sticking in the lungs causing cancer in a similar way that asbestos causes mesothelioma. Using Electron Microscopy, silver nanoparticles are measured to be 20-30 nm and does not fit in the alleged size parameter.

In a publication on H5N1 bird flu[44] a specific brand of silver was used to help prevent the bird flu and a simultaneous toxicity study was performed wherein 10 times normal, 100 times normal, and 200 times normal amounts of the liquid silver supplement were given to mice. Lung necropsy was performed to determine if the lung tissues were damaged. It was found that the lung tissues had reduced viral titers, were less inflamed and weighed less, indicating that the lungs were not being harmed by nanoparticles. In addition the lower lung weights indicate that there was a reduction in the inflammation supporting the safety of the particle. Structured silver is alkaline and promotes better healing potentials than the form of silver used in the above study.

Ingesting Silver is Normal

For the internal use of silver, many people feel nervous about swallowing it until they realize that they already do it every day.

Silver is ingested in many foods. Mushrooms contain silver concentrations as high as several hundred parts per billion. Most meats contain silver. According to World Health Organization estimates, people typically consume between 20 and 50 micrograms of silver on a daily basis.

Not surprisingly, silver is found in our bodily tissues. One of the highest concentrations of silver is within the platelets of our blood. This is interesting, as platelets are an essential part of the body's natural healing response.

Silver is also found in our drinking water, lakes and rivers. The EPA suggests that drinking water should contain less that 0.10 milligrams per liter of water [45], which translates roughly into 0.1 ppm. Note that this is for daily drinking water, which is measured in liters, whereas a 10 ppm silver supplement is taken only teaspoons at a time. The silver within structured silver is prepared for optimal benefit and does not require a high concentration.

Although we encounter silver on a daily basis through our diets and environment, not all forms of silver are the same. Some forms of silver can be poisonous, such as silver proteins, silver salts and industrial byproducts containing silver. It is important to distinguish products containing silver from one another. Always ask yourself, "Which form of silver is it?"

Preventative

As a result of its safety, a pH-balanced silver can be used as a full-time preventive antimicrobial. It is excreted so quickly and thoroughly that regular small ingestions (two teaspoons twice daily) are typically recommended for general usage. Most silver products are acids and can cause caustic burns inside or outside the body. Why use the acidic form of silver when there is an alkaline silver?

Alkaline silver works with the immune system while acids trigger immune cascades of mobilized and activated immune cells that cause swelling, inflammation and even autoimmunity, frequently preventing the daily use of acidic silver. Alkaline silver works with the immune system promoting healing by destroying the pathogens without abnormal immune swelling and inflammation. For this and other reasons the alkaline or pH balanced silver can be taken every day.

Unlike conventional antibiotics, which are only available by prescription and are typically not recommended for long-term use, structured silver is able to combat pathogens without creating resistance. This can be helpful for general use, for protection when traveling, or for preventive use when visiting places with an elevated risk of infection.

For topical applications such as facial cleansing, hand disinfection, or vaginal cleansing daily use of a gel is also safe.

Structured Silver Passes From the Body Unmetabolized

Not many substances pass through the body unmetabolized (a scientist's way of saying "it doesn't change between swallowing and excretion"), but structured silver does just that. This is an unusual characteristic for an antimicrobial. Pharmaceutical products that work by chemical action are typically consumed while killing germs within the body, one molecule at a time, until the dose is fully utilized. In contrast, structured silver liquid's ability to work by physics without chemical consumption is a distinguishing characteristic that is surprising to those of the biochemistry paradigm.

The result is that structured silver is just as effective at disinfecting when it is leaving the body (killing the germs that cause bladder infections and urinary tract infections) as it was when it was swished in the mouth several hours earlier (killing the germs that cause gum disease, bad breath, cold sores, etc.) In between drinking and excretion, it will have been equally effective while circulating through the bloodstream (killing pathogens wherever the blood flows) or traveling through the digestive tract (killing pathogens like E. coli or Salmonella a person may have swallowed at lunchtime).

For women who experience frequent bladder and urinary tract infections, this is welcome news. As urine gathers in the bladder and is excreted, the same silver that eliminated germs throughout the body will disinfect the organs of excretion as well.

Topical Use

While structured silver is effective for internal cleansing, it is equally effective on the surface of the body. For example, pathogens can flourish on the skin within wrinkles, scrapes, pores, bites, cuticles, piercings, and even burns such as sunburn. Prevention of small external infections can have a rapid effect. pH-balanced structured silver can be applied topically as a gel and as a liquid using a mister, gauze, or soaking the skin.

Structured silver makes a perfect skin conditioner because it does not contain alcohol or petroleum products. Alcohol can dry the skin, which can cause cracking and bleeding when used consistently. Petroleum-based sanitizers can leave a greasy residue, causing a tacky feeling or flakes once the product has dried. When alkaline silver is combined with aloe vera in a gel the skin responds without irritation and becomes moist and sustains it for a longer time. This is significant to the healing process as a moist wound or skin repairs itself best. Wet or dry skin leave scars or don't close. The combination of aloe as a moisturizer and silver makes a perfect all natural anti-aging formula.

Skin can be damaged by many things, including wind, sun, makeup, and detergent. The protective barrier that usually keeps our skin healthy comes from oils that are secreted by the skin, but as we get older we secrete less and less of these protective oils. By using a silver gel on the skin one to four times a day, the skin will stay moist and a protective antibacterial barrier will be created to prevent disease from entering the skin.

The gel can also be combined with other routines and products on a daily basis. For example, silver gel combined with aloe provides a moisturizing benefit that protects and promotes skin health. Skin needs to be moist to avoid premature aging; by destroying the pathogens that cause thick scarred and damaged tissues at the same time you receive the benefits of healing, softness and smoothness. For additional skin supplementation, amino acids, vitamin E, or flax oil supplements can be helpful.

General Uses for Body Systems

Structured silver may be your most effective tool to maintain, sustain and support your immune defenses. This chapter provides basic guidelines for appropriate application of structured silver depending on how it is being used. More detailed information on specific health challenges is given in a later chapter.

An important question to ask with your healthcare professional is, "if there are pathogens in the body that structured silver can kill on contact, how do I get the right amount of silver to specific locations around the body?" This is basically a question of delivery. Since the body is complex, different delivery strategies are needed for different parts of the body and for different infections.

Here are several recommendations, organized by body system.

General Usage:

· Maintenance dose: 2 teaspoons, hold under tongue for 30 seconds then swallow, twice a day
· Acute Immune Issue: 2 tablespoons 2-3 times a day

Respiratory System:

· Respiratory Health: Swallow two teaspoons twice daily and spray 3-4 sprays in nose as needed.
· Nasal Health / Allergies: Swallow 2 teaspoons twice daily and spray into the nose 3-4 sprays 4 times a day.
· Mouth and Gum Health: Twice daily, hold 2 tablespoons in mouth and gargle for 4-5 minutes, then swallow.
· Throat Health: Hold 2 tablespoons in mouth for 3 minutes then swallow; repeat several times a day. If using spray, 15 sprays every other hour.
· Lung Health: Swallow 2 tablespoons 2-3 times a day, and inhale 4 sprays four times a day.

Cardiovascular Health:

· 2 tablespoons, hold in mouth for 1 minute, then swallow, twice a day.

Digestive / Intestinal System:

· Gastrointestinal Health: Swallow two teaspoons twice daily.
· Intestinal Health Balance: Take 2 tablespoons of silver 2-3 times a day and

combine with probiotics twice a day.

Urinary System:

· Drink 2 tablespoons twice daily.

Female Specific:

· Female Health: Use two to three ounces in affected area, hold for ten minutes then release, 1-2 times daily. And drink 2 tablespoons twice daily.

Sensory System:

· Ear Health: Point ear towards the sky and put 5 drops into ear and hold upright for 10 minutes. Repeat every 12 hours. And swallow 2 teaspoons twice daily.
· Eye Health: Use 1-2 drops every hour.

Immune/Allergy Health:

· Nasal Health / Allergies: Swallow 2 teaspoons twice daily and spray into the nose 3-4 sprays 1-4 times a day.

First Aid Recovery Support for Cuts, Scrapes, Bug Bites, etc.:

· To support the immune system, swallow 2 teaspoons twice a day and apply gel topically as needed.

Skin and Nails:

· Skin Health: To support the immune system, apply gel twice daily or as needed, and swallow liquid 2 teaspoons twice daily.
· Nail Fungus: Frequent use of small amounts of product is best.

Healthy Water:

· 2 tablespoons per gallon of water, wait 4 minutes, drink as needed.

Traveling

· Swallow 2 teaspoons before, during and after flying or driving, for general immune support. Hold under tongue for 30 seconds before swallowing. And spray.
· 3-4 sprays into nose before flying.

Please be aware that federal regulations limit dietary supplements to oral administration even if structure function claims may be specific to certain body parts.

Immune System

Structured silver is a mild immune modulator. It has been shown to cause an increase in the number and activity of immune cells when taken orally. This means that if you drink a teaspoon of silver liquid twice daily you will find an increase in the number of white blood cells, which destroy foreign pathogens in the body. It should be noted that this improvement in immune health occurs within an hour after drinking silver and will last for approximately 24-48 hours after. You can expect to have improved defenses against bacteria viruses and yeast during the time you are taking a structured silver and for a day or two after. In addition silver can help protect and shield the body from diseases caused by these pathogens by killing them upon direct contact.

Recommendations:

Drink one teaspoon 2 times daily to support immune function, and apply a pH-balanced silver gel as needed to affected areas that require gel application. Benefits can be measured in the blood within one hour and will last up to two days after the last drink. Benefits from the gel can be felt in 3-5 minutes as it helps reduce pain and inflammation. For more serious health concerns silver liquid can be taken 2-4 times greater doses.

Respiratory System

Structured silver destroys bacteria viruses and yeast that resides in or around the respiratory system (ears, nose, throat, lungs).

Recommendations:

- Inhaled (from a nebulizer 30 minutes a day or two episodes of 15 minutes each).
- Drink two teaspoons twice a day, or spray fine mist up nose 2-5 times a day.
- Apply gel to the nose, sinuses mouth, and hands to prevent infections or spread of germs. This can be done 1-5 times a day or as often as it keeps the nasal passages moist.

Reproductive System

Silver benefits the reproductive organs by destroying bacteria, viruses and yeast that may cause damage to the delicate organs and tissues of the reproductive system.

Silver destroys bacteria that cause urinary tract infections and yeast that causes yeast infections. This can be accomplished in about ten minutes as long as the silver comes in close proximity to the germs.

Recommendations:

· Drink liquid silver two teaspoons twice a day to help destroy germs from the inside out.

· Apply silver gel to the reproductive tissues that are susceptible to infections (vagina, penis, foreskin, breast, pubic hair etc.). This should be done twice a day or more often if needed.

· Apply the silver gel to a tampon and insert for 90 minutes in order to stay in contact with germs intravaginally.

· Apply the gel twice a day to the foreskin, condom or genitals to protect yourself or your sex partner.

Circulatory System

Structured silver destroys the bacterium that causes cardiovascular diseases. The gel can be used as toothpaste to kill the bacteria that causes bad breath, cavities, abscesses, and heart disease because this kind of bacteria resides in the gums. A mouthwash twice a day will kill bacteria in the mouth as well.

Digestive System

Silver liquid and gel can be swallowed and enter the digestive tract where it will destroy bacteria, viruses and yeast. There are serious diseases that originate in the intestines, colon, and vital organs of digestion. Silver can pass through the digestive tract unchanged. This means the silver kills germs in the kidneys and bladder just as effectively as it kills bacteria in the mouth. This is significant because kidney, liver and bladder infections are very difficult to control but silver will pass through the bloodstream and flow through the liver, thus cleansing the germs out of the liver, then pass through the kidneys and on to the bladder where pathogens will be destroyed when they come in close proximity with the silver nanoparticles.

Recommendations:

· Drink two teaspoons of silver liquid twice daily for digestive health. In the event there is a food poisoning, diarrhea, or other digestive malady, silver liquid can be swallowed one ounce every hour for 12 hours or until remedied. Usually the most serious symptoms of the food poisoning problem can be brought under control in 2-4 hours with the remainder of the sickness requiring maintenance doses (two teaspoons twice daily).

· Apply the gel to any orifice of the body that may need protection from germs (1-4 times a day).

Hair Skin and Nails

Structured silver liquid and gel destroys the bacteria, viruses and yeast that cause diseases in the hair, skin and nails. The liquid can be used in shampoo, lotions, gels, and moisturizers and under nails. The gel can be applied to all skin conditions and can be pushed under nails to destroy yeast.

Recommendations:

· All of these can benefit from drinking structured silver liquid two teaspoons twice a day and applying the gel 2-4 times a day or as needed topically.

The ESSENCE of Wellness

Structured silver should be used as one part of a broader commitment to good health and wellness. Silver's benefits and effects are enhanced dramatically by what I call the ESSENCE of health. Each letter in the word determines one healthy principle.

E - eat correctly
S - sleep enough
S - supplement
E - exercise more
N - neutralize toxins
C - cleanse regularly
E - eliminate stress

If you perform one of these essential values you will receive a certain level of protection from disease and degeneration. However, by combining multiple values, your ability to prevent disease and promote wellness increases exponentially.

Exponential Benefit

In my dissertation research I examined exercise, nutrition, and the combination of both in preventing fatal viral infections. I discovered different types of exercise mobilize and activate the immune system, resulting in a 16 percent increase in immune cells. I also measured an 18 percent increase in the activity of immune cells (NK cells) due to herbal supplementation.

These benefits help a person function optimally and feel better. However, when a person exercised and took nutritional supplementation at the same time, they received an exponential increase in the number and activity of immune cells. When the protective levels of exercise were combined with the protective levels of nutritional supplementation, there was a 255 percent increase in the NK cells. These are the immune cells responsible for killing all foreign pathogens, including fatal viruses and cancers.

I then combined exercise and nutritional supplementation together with a fatal virus (Cytomegalovirus CMV) to see if mice were able to prevent or survive a fatal viral challenge. Again, the principles of wellness were proven beneficial as the infected mice, which exercised on a treadmill and were fed nutritional supplements, survived a fatal viral infection. This experiment resulted in a 56 percent increase in the ability to survive a fatal viral infection, just by walking and taking nutritional supplements.

This example demonstrates how every healthy tool you give your body is one more level of protection. Adding multiple layers of protection increases your ability to prevent disease and promote wellness.

Commitment to Good Health

A few years ago a chairperson for the National Institutes of Health's Antiviral Committee, Dr. Sidwell, caught a sinus infection that lingered for weeks and kept getting worse. He felt horrible—headaches, pain, fatigue, and sinuses that just wouldn't drain.

He went to his doctor and started antibiotics, and when they didn't work he started a stronger combination of antibiotics. That didn't work either, so he started using the antiviral drugs he had developed. After some lab work it was determined that his sinus infection was resistant to all drugs. His doctor suggested surgery to keep the infection from going into his ears, eyes, and brain.

This was enough to scare him. At the time I was not aware of silver and its many benefits, so I had suggested herbal supplements, exercise, and a good sleep system. He was not inclined to act until he heard the word "surgery." He took the herbs, rode a bike, and got some rest. Within three days his sinuses were completely clear— without the aid of drugs!

He was amazed. After all, he was the inventor of antiviral drugs, and yet he avoided surgery with just supplements and exercise. All his years of wisdom convinced him that prevention was still the best answer. He continues to take supplements, exercise, and has water and air filters in his home.

From this experience I learned that, in addition to the above measures, family support has a profound impact on health. Dr. Sidwell is my father-in-law. It is scary to think that without his wife and children encouraging him to stick to a health regimen, the results may have been different. Fortunately, his family was firmly committed to the essence of good health.

Let's take a closer look at what it means to follow the ESSENCE of good health.

E: Eat Correctly

The U.S. Department of Agriculture reports that 92 percent of Americans do not get sufficient nutrients from the foods they eat. Their dietary guidelines include balancing diet with exercise, eating grains with fruits and vegetables, eating a low-fat diet, choosing a diet low in sugars, salt and alcohol, and not smoking or using tobacco.

To meet these guidelines, supplementation is needed—especially for children and the elderly. A child who doesn't receive proper nutrition will not achieve maximum physical and mental potential. The immune systems will not function correctly, bones don't grow properly and muscles are weak.

Most children develop their eating habits in the home and have established their eating and exercise habits by age 15. A recent report claims Americans are drinking more soda and eating less fresh whole foods. Those habits can carry on into later years. Here are the results from a recent survey of college students:

· 15 percent of college students did not eat any vegetables
· 40 percent ate a diet high in foods like French fries and ketchup, which they consider to be healthy forms of potatoes and tomatoes
· 20 percent did not consume any fruit

During the four years of college, the average girl gains 20 pounds. This diet shows one reason why. It has been reported that in the year 1900 the average person consumed 6-8 pounds of sugar per year. Today the estimate is over 200 pounds of sugar—and 1 in 13 adults are becoming diabetic in the process!

Conversely, there are tremendous benefits for those who consume natural fruit nectars and green drinks, eat vegetables, and keep sugar to a minimum. Adding fresh food to your diet provides antioxidants that neutralize toxins.

It is important to eat organic produce. Our fruits and vegetables are irradiated with up to 30 million x-rays to stop the enzymes from softening fresh fruit. Genetically-altered fruits and vegetables can be detrimental to our health.

S: Sleep Enough

Sleep deprivation costs America an estimated 100 billion dollars a year in lost productivity, medical expenses, and sick leave time.

A National Sleep Foundation poll found the following:

- Nearly 7 out of 10 Americans said they experience sleep problems
- 69 percent of children have a sleep problem at least once a week
- 67 percent of elderly adults (40 and older) report frequent sleep problems
- 63 percent of adults do not get 8 hours of sleep a night (adults need 7-9 hours of sleep per night)
- 15 percent of adults have severe insomnia

When we don't get adequate sleep, we accumulate a sleep debt that can be difficult to pay back. If our sleep debt gets too high, we start to experience physical, emotional, and hormonal damage, including high blood pressure, obesity, and mood and behavior changes.

In a study, 20-year-olds were only allowed to sleep four hours a night for seven days. At the end of the week they all tested positive for diabetes or hypoglycemia. This shows that lack of sleep can cause hormones to change.

How can you increase and improve your sleep? Exercise during the day helps exhaust your excess physical stress. A good diet can help you get better quality sleep, which helps you feel better rested in the morning. Even a simple back massage can help relax the muscles and make going to sleep easier.

A schoolteacher and mother of four children didn't get more than five hours of sleep a night. Her family insisted something was wrong because she continued to gain weight, even when she ate half-meals. While visiting the doctor, she found she was insulin resistant and diabetic.

Her chiropractor recommended she take supplements, sleep 8 hours a night and walk 20 minutes every day. She was miraculously able to control her insulin levels without continued insulin injection, and within a year she lost 35 pounds.

S: Supplement

As mentioned earlier, 92 percent of Americans do not get what they need from the foods they eat. There are more than 20,000 medical journal articles demonstrating the benefits of nutritional supplements. Even U.S. Public Law 103-417 states that the use of dietary supplements will prevent disease, promote wellness, and reduce long-term health care costs.

Structured silver can be combined with any nutritional supplement, from herbs and antibiotics to pharmaceutical drugs. It should not, however, be combined with salt, as the chloride ion inactivates some of silver's effectiveness. After eating salty foods, wait one hour before using silver.

As detailed in the following section (EXERCISE MORE), supplementation can exponentially increase the effects of exercise and healthy living. Supplements can also benefit specific body systems such as gastrointestinal, immune, respiratory, and circulatory.

E: Exercise More

According to Health and Hygiene Journal, exercise helps prevent coronary heart disease, stroke, and some forms of cancer. Unfortunately, 6 out of 10 men and 7 out of 10 women are not sufficiently active to benefit their health, according to the Department of Health and CDC.

The average American has been gaining three pounds per year since the 1980s. More than 65 percent of us are overweight and 31 percent are obese, often due to lack of exercise and poor diet. The U.S. Health and Human Services Committee reports that obesity is the second leading cause of preventable death, with more than 300,000 obesity-related deaths each year.

The best solution for all of these problems is to walk 90 minutes a week. I recommend walking with weighted shoes, as it helps your legs grow stronger and helps you get exercise no matter what you're doing. If you walk five days a week you can realistically expect to burn 25 pounds of fat during the year.

I conducted research on the benefits of exercise in combination with nutritional supplements. Here's what I found:

By walking daily, you can increase the number of immune NK cells by about 15 percent. If you sprint for 10 seconds you can increase immune cells by about 23 percent. If you alternately walk and jog, you get about an 18 percent increase. This benefit lasts about four hours and offers added protection against viruses and abnormal cell growth.

I also tested what would happen if you only used a nutritional supplement and found that the activity of the immune cell increased by 18 percent. I found it remarkable that a supplement would activate the immune system.

I then combined exercise with nutritional supplementation and discovered a 255 percent increase in the number of NK cells. They continued to be active for 20 hours.

When you combine exercise with supplements you get an exponential benefit to the immune system that lasts five times longer. You should note that these are the immune cells that fight viruses and cancers best.

I wanted to see if this would prevent a fatal viral infection like the flu. When I infected mice with a fatal virus and then gave them supplements and exercised them on a treadmill, they developed a 64 percent increase in the ability to survive a fatal viral infection.

Here's the most important thing I learned from this process—exercise results in a mild benefit and supplement use results in a mild benefit. But when you combine the two, you increase the ability to fight off disease exponentially.

In addition to its benefit to the immune system, a new study also reports the benefits of exercise on depression. Those who exercised 90 minutes a week over a two-and-a-half month period were better able to control their depression more than by using tricyclic antidepressants (such as Prozac).

N: Neutralize Toxins in the Air and Water

The adult body is about 60 percent water and that of a child is 75 percent water. By the time we feel thirsty we are already dehydrated. Dehydration can cause dizziness, headache, dry mouth and tongue, confusion and incoherence. It is also the leading cause of hospitalization in those over 65.

To stay adequately hydrated, you must drink about 8 glasses of water per day. By drinking clean, pure water you can also help avoid excess body fat, poor muscle tone, constipation, toxic overload, and joint and muscle soreness.

Proper fluid intake is also a major key to weight loss. If you are dehydrated you will not lose fat. In fact, it takes 22 ounces of water to metabolize one ounce of fat. No water means no fat burning as your body is forced to use muscle for energy and to store fat.

Most of us don't realize that 90 percent of the time we think we are hungry, we are really just thirsty. The next time you are hungry in between meals, drink eight ounces of clean, pure water and wait 15 minutes. This will often curb your hunger.

Water Toxins

In America, 178 million people get their water from surface water systems and 85.9 million get it from ground water systems. This means that two thirds of Americans are really drinking water that was collected from the surface, i.e., the gutter. Forty percent of America is drinking water that is potentially unfit to drink!

Water helps convert food into energy. It also regulates body temperature; moistens the mouth, eyes and nose; and removes toxins through proper excretion. Contaminated water fills our bodies with toxins and can cause major diseases.

We should always try to drink optimized water. "Optimized" means that one oxygen molecule is combined with two hydrogen molecules and can transfer energy readily. The problem is that in tap water, for every one oxygen molecule, there are usually 36 hydrogen molecules clinging on and becoming free radicals once ingested.

Air Toxins

We spend 90 percent of our time inside. The EPA reports that 6 out of 10 buildings are contaminated with air pollution. These buildings can be 100 times more toxic than outdoor air. Toxins from carpet chemicals, cleansers, paint, glue, dust, and mold accumulate in your lungs, stick in your

NINE REASONS TO DRINK CLEAN, PURE, OPTIMIZED WATER:

1. 75 percent of Americans are regularly dehydrated

2. 37 percent believe they are hungry when they are really thirsty because of toxins

3. A 3 percent dehydration results in slow metabolism (which means weight gain)

4. A 2 percent loss of body water results in short-term memory loss and trouble focusing

5. Children who don't absorb enough water are linked to obesity and reduced height

6. Water reduces cramps, fevers, and the craving for sweets

alveoli, and never come out again.

Some big cities have traffic and smog so thick it burns the eyes and clogs the lungs and skin pores. If you can smell the pollution in your hair as you wash it, just imagine the impact it is having on your lungs.

The Centers for Disease Control (CDC) recommends HEPA filters to remove bacteria and viruses. These filters are used in hospitals to keep doctors healthy despite being exposed to so many unhealthy people. These filters are especially beneficial in the winter months when bacteria spread is rampant.

C: Cleanse

A clean home is a healthy home. This is the case for the human body as well. It requires regular cleansing of the intestines, blood, liver, and other vital organs. When the body is not clean, diseases begin to damage healthy tissues until eventually the systems of the body fail.

If you build a new wall over a wet and dirty area, mold can grow and eat away the newly formed walls. This is true with the intestinal system as well. If a person has a clogged intestine (constipation), no good thing can be absorbed. This leads to intestinal molds, yeasts, and other pathogens that damage the intestines and detoxification organs. When the intestines can't detoxify the fermenting foods fast enough, the extra burden falls on the liver and kidneys. These vital organs can perform very well, but only for a limited time. If the constipation continues, diseases can develop from chronic exposure to intestinal toxins.

With an intestinal cleanse, the body will be able to eliminate toxins from all systems of the body, including the brain. Without a regular cleanse, detoxification organs are overworked. Fermented sugars are stored in the muscles and the bloodstream begins to circulate potentially pathogenic elements to all parts of the body.

No system of your body will work optimally if it is not cleansed regularly. You will heal faster, more completely, and with less inflammation if you consistently cleanse your intestines, blood, and liver.

E: Eliminate Stress

The word stress comes from the Latin strigi, which means, "to be drawn tight." Anyone who has experienced stress knows this is a very apt description.

There are four types of stress: eustress (good), distress (bad), hyperstress (too much), and hypostress (not enough). Regardless of the type, stress produces physical, psychological, emotional, and behavioral symptoms, including:

- Racing heart
- Breathlessness
- Tight chest
- Dry mouth
- Indigestion
- Muscle twitches
- Frequent attacks of flu and sore throat (compromised immune system)
- Indecisiveness
- Poor concentration
- Bad dreams
- Sexual dysfunction
- Negative thoughts (including thoughts of suicide)
- Irritability
- Sleep disturbances
- Anger
- Blood sugar imbalances
- Low self-esteem
- Neglected self-care
- Tendency to avoid social activities
- Substance abuse
- Depression
- Lack of confidence

Stress is worse than you may think. In fact, some doctors believe stress is the major cause of all disease. It tears away at every body system, including your brain. Even worse, the stress of your past experiences also magnifies your reactivity to stress in the future.

Stress has a central command post—the hypothalamus, which regulates heart rate, blood pressure, and all involuntary bodily functions. Under long or extreme stress, the brain and its chemistry change, resulting in long- and short-term changes to behavior, personality and even memory. Stress lowers natural immunity and allows damage to tissues, resulting in diseases such as rheumatoid arthritis and fibromyalgia. Stress also makes it hard to lose weight.

Fortunately, stress can be reduced and prevented and the symptoms can be reversed over time. A drink comprised of whole fruits can be used to protect the cellular DNA that might be damaged by cortisol. A supplement of omega-3 fatty acids can protect the hypothalamus in the brain from becoming overworked, confused, or shutting down. A green drink can reduce the toxins from stress by helping them leave through the colon quickly. Each of these products contains antioxidants and can help reduce free radicals. When I travel to foreign countries, I experience jet lag and stress. I always try to sleep 12 hours and have a green drink to get me jump-started again.

Winning the War

The fight against disease is not a lost cause. I feel strongly that by combining healthy habits of ESSENCE with regular use of structured silver, the vast majority of contagious disease can be prevented and we can win the war.

E - eat correctly
S - sleep enough
S - supplement
E - exercise more
N - neutralize toxins
C - cleanse regularly
E - eliminate stress

Let's now take a look at the wide range of silver uses.

Silver Uses A-Z

This chapter provides information for people with specific health challenges in mind. In the general rule of thumb is "two teaspoons twice per day; apply gel as needed." This chapter is a detailed list of exceptions and additions.

Abscesses

Because it's an open wound, an abscess can expose the blood flow to possible bacterial contamination. It is very important to kill the bacteria in the wound.

An alkaline structured silver can be used as a mouth rinse for an abscess in the mouth. Hold one ounce of liquid in your mouth for at least six minutes, two to three times a day. It can then be swallowed, providing an internal rinse as well.

You can also use liquid silver as a rinse for an abscess on the outside of your body. When you first clean the abscess, rinse it with silver liquid. If it requires a bandage, soak the gauze bandage in liquid structured silver and put a drop of gel on the surface before taping it into place.

For a very small abscess, you can simply put a drop of the silver gel on a Band-Aid and place it over the abscess. For a large abscess, spray the gel or the liquid silver on the wound one to four times a day.

Aches

Aches can occur from inflammation within a joint, muscle, or body system, like the intestinal or cardiovascular system. Structured silver has the ability to destroy the cause of inflammation—bacteria, viruses, parasites, and even yeast in some cases.

By killing the cause, inflammation can be reduced, maintained, and even prevented. Just take one teaspoon of structured silver one to three times a day. Using glucosamine, chondroitin sulfate, and MSM also helps aches. In addition, silver has the ability to help modulate the cause of pain in a very mild manner.

Acid Reflux

Acid reflux is also referred to as heartburn. It occurs when too much stomach acid pools in the stomach and then returns back into the throat or mouth. The associated pain is a result of the hydrochloric acid dissolving and digesting the normal tissues of the esophagus, mouth, and throat.

To stop the problem, it is necessary to stop the flow of acid. One way is to take digestive enzymes and neutralize those acids. Another way is to take antacids, which help absorb those acids and pass them through your digestive tract.

Structured silver can be taken daily to help the burns caused by the acid. Take one to two teaspoons, two to five times a day as needed. In addition, you can take acidophilus or digestive enzymes, which help transport stomach acids out of the body. As a last resort, a physician can prescribe acid blockers or drugs that will stop the production of acid in the stomach.

A young woman in her early 20s was taken to the emergency room, thinking she might be having a heart attack. After being checked for all the signs and symptoms, a heart attack was ruled out. Yet she was still doubled over in pain and having stabbing pains right over her heart. She was given a cocktail of antacids and pain relievers, and within a few minutes the pain subsided. The doctors deduced that it was not a heart attack, but acid reflux.

Two weeks later she was in the same situation, experiencing the same stabbing pain. Because she knew it was acid reflux, she went to the store and bought over-the-counter acid blockers. This worked for about six months.

She had to keep increasing the quantity and frequency of her acid blocker use to find relief. She soon noticed a sore throat that she just couldn't get rid of. It became so bothersome that she went back to the doctor.

The doctor found that her sore throat was caused by acid reflux. The acid had been traveling from her stomach up to her throat, literally dissolving the back of her throat. Acid reflux is strong enough to dissolve your esophagus to the point that surgery is needed to repair the damage. Luckily she caught it in time.

This young woman also had a lot of fever blisters. When she would lie down at night, the acid would reflux up her esophagus and into her mouth. The acid would start to burn little holes in her mouth and cause cankers. If you frequently have cankers, it may be from acid reflux. To find relief, you should utilize silver, digestive enzymes, and acidophilus on a regular basis.

Acne

Acne attacks people of all ages, from infants to adults. Bacteria getting inside of a hair follicle or a sweat gland called a sebaceous gland can cause acne. Once the bacteria gets under the skin it will duplicate itself, dissolving healthy tissue in the process and leaving scars behind. To get rid of the acne, you must get rid of the bacteria.

To kill the bacteria, take two teaspoons of silver twice a day. Silver gel should also be applied topically twice a day.

You can expect to see reduction in the size and in the damage of the acne within 24 hours. Total improvement of the skin will take about four weeks—the amount of time necessary for new skin to grow from the bottom to the top layer.

Antibiotics and Silver

Dr. Rustum Roy published an article in the medical journal Current Science about silver. His findings showed silver can improve healing functions because it is a broad-spectrum microbial, similar in results to any pharmaceutical-grade antibiotic—without causing resistance, mutation, or tolerance like antibiotics.

An antibiotic can only be taken for about two weeks before bacteria mutate and become resistant to the drug. For this reason, antibiotics can't be used on a continuous basis for prevention. A pH-balanced structured silver creates no resistance. It is alkaline so it can be taken every day without fear of disrupting your body's pH. In addition, antibiotics only work on a narrow range of bacteria; silver has a very broad range of use.

When antibiotics are supplemented with structured silver the benefits can be as much as tenfold. Use silver daily for prevention. If a crisis occurs, antibiotics can be added. The silver will destroy the bacteria that the antibiotic misses.

ADD - Attention Deficit Disorder

Though we are unsure of all the causes and types of Attention Deficit Disorder (ADD), we do know that sugar can be a trigger and certain drugs, vaccinations, and lack of sleep may all play a role as well.

In the event of ADD, it is important to reduce sugar, cleanse the intestinal system, and restore proper function to the brain with B-vitamins, lecithin, phosphatidyl serine, and essential fatty acids. Drinking two teaspoons of structured silver twice a day will kill bacteria, viruses, and mold, and reduce the neurotoxins sent to the brain.

Age Spots

Age spots develop when the liver doesn't produce enough enzymes to detoxify what is circulating through the bloodstream. Certain toxins can be deposited in the fats underneath your skin, creating an age spot—usually a permanent effect like a tattoo.

You can get the liver working properly again, and get the proper production of enzymes at the same time, by drinking liquid structured silver on a regular basis. Putting silver gel on the age spot can help reduce that which has been stored under the skin. For the best benefit, apply topically two to four times a day and take one teaspoon orally twice a day.

Aging

There are many reasons why we may age prematurely—a liver that doesn't function properly, tissues that degenerate too quickly, a sedentary lifestyle, lack of nutrients, and the toxins that are all around us.

Yeast is one of the main components in premature aging. We have yeast between our toes and in our intestines. It's found anywhere there is a warm, moist area and destroys one cell at a time. Likewise, bacteria can cause tissue damage. Silver prevents premature aging by killing bacteria, viruses, and yeast.

Drink one teaspoon of a liquid pH–balanced silver twice a day for wellness and prevention. If you are sick, drink two teaspoons twice a day. Silver gel can also be applied to specific areas topically one to three times a day. Additional benefits can come from using freeform amino acids, vitamins, minerals, and essential fatty acids.

A research project was conducted to see if structured silver could help prevent aging in roses. Eighteen roses were clipped from the same bush. The leaves were stripped off and each rose was placed in its own vase. Each vase contained water; half of the vases also contained structured silver liquid.

The roses placed only in water died in a week and a half. The roses supplemented with structured silver were in bloom and fully healthy for three and a half weeks. Structured silver helped prolong the life of a rose by at least 200%. And surprisingly, the roses in the structured silver liquid regrew their leaves. Silver not only helped prevent the aging process from taking place, it demonstrated regenerative properties with new leaves growing where the old leaves had been stripped off.

Allergies

Allergies occur when an allergen triggers an allergic response in the body. The immune system mobilizes and activates, causing inflammation, swelling, and mucus

My mother suffers from allergies in her ears, nose and throat. When the season changes to winter and the heater turns on and the air dries out, so do her sinuses. The physicians want to give her decongestants and antibiotics, but this produces more problems in her digestive and immune systems. Instead she drinks one ounce of silver liquid twice a day and sprays a mist of silver liquid up her nose as needed to keep the cause of congestion under control.

In addition she puts silver liquid into her ultrasonic humidifier and lets the mist spray over her during sleep. By using a humidifier in the room, it helps her sinuses stay moist. Dry sinuses crack and bleed, allowing germs to grow in clogged and swollen sinus cavities. In addition, she uses a few drops of structured silver in her ears if they become irritated. The message is that silver can help prevent infections in the ears, sinus, throat, and lungs.

production. When this happens in the throat or the sinuses, it results in a sore throat or sinus infection. This can lead to coughing, sneezing, irritation in our lungs and even asthma-like symptoms.

The first step to improving asthma symptoms is to remove the allergen—e.g., the pollen, the dust, or irritating laundry detergent. While we can't remove all the allergens from our air or water, we can remove a lot of bacteria, viruses, and mold from inside our body by drinking liquid structured silver. We can protect the outside of our body by using silver gel topically.

To fight allergies, drink one teaspoon in the morning and one at night. Spraying silver into the nasal cavities will also reduce swelling and congestion. Nebulized silver can be inhaled a total of 30 minutes each day and gel can be applied inside the nostrils to counteract skin irritation.

Alzheimer's Disease

Alzheimer's disease causes the brain to slowly lose function. There are many suspected causes, from heavy metal toxicity to inflammation. According to the MERK Index medical journal, silver is the one metal that is not classified as a heavy metal. It will not accumulate in the brain like lead does. In fact, structured silver has been used in combination with freeform amino acids and phosphatidyl serine to help improve circulation and mental memory and function. Taking one teaspoon of structured silver morning and evening will destroy intestinal neurotoxins that cause inflammation of the brain.

Antibacterial

Found on the skin, in the bloodstream, in the intestines, or in the hair, bacteria cause countless diseases. When serious diseases are examined in the lab they find that every serious chronic disease is associated with the presence of pleiomorphic bacteria or mold. These damage the immune function that normally protects the cell from foreign invaders. When the bacteria or mold invade a cell and reduce the immune protection, they allow toxins and contagions to enter the cell and damage the DNA, allowing serious disease to originate. Structured silver starts killing bacteria in as little as fifteen seconds. If you put structured silver gel, liquid, or mist in direct contact with bacteria, the bacteria will usually be totally destroyed within six minutes. Some bacteria may take longer but can be destroyed with regular structured silver use.

For preventive use, drink one teaspoon of silver liquid each morning and night. That dose can be doubled to fight an aggressive bacterial infection. Silver gel may be applied topically to any affected areas one to four times a day. Immune-supporting herbs may also be used.

Nursing home residents often have a weakened immune system. This makes them susceptible to bacterial infections. Many develop bedsores, and bacteria—like staph—will get into the sore. Bedsores can last up to seven years without healing. Imagine having an open wound, living in a nursing home, and having an infection that is treated with antibiotics that stop working after just a few weeks.

Structured silver gel is currently being used in clinical trials. Results are showing that it can help close deep open-tunneling wounds, leprosy, and staph, including MRSA. By spraying the gel on the wound twice a day, bacteria are destroyed and the body can heal itself more quickly.

Anti-fungal

Fungus can get into any warm, moist area and often feeds off of sugars. Cutting off sugars can combat intestinal fungus or yeast. For a yeast or fungus infection in the armpits or vagina, apply silver gel directly to the yeast or take liquid structured silver internally. It can be applied topically one to four times a day, or as needed. The recommend liquid use is two teaspoons, one to three times a day. Acidophilus supplementation may be used simultaneously.

Yeast and fungus can get inside your intestines, causing muscle pain and symptoms of depression and attention deficit disorder. It can also result in all the symptoms of headaches, lymph problems, lupus and autoimmune disorders, including fibromyalgia.

Many people have resolved these symptoms by taking two teaspoons of a structured silver daily as part of an intestinal yeast and fungus cleanse. The cleanse may be accompanied by one to three weeks of flu-like symptoms while the yeast leaves the body. Structured silver colonics have been used in the rectum, and douches are being successful used in the vagina.

Anti-Tumor

Tumors can have a myriad of causes. Tumors are almost always caused by a combination of problems. One bacterium is not usually the cause of a tumor, but when bacteria get into the cell and neutralize your immune function, you become more susceptible to other toxins in the air and water. This allows DNA to be damaged and a tumor to form. Bacteria such as hepatitis B can cause cancer. Viruses can also cause tumors and cancer, including the human papilloma virus that can result in cervical cancer in women.

Those with a tumor should drink one to four ounces of structured silver liquid a day, sipping the structured silver every hour for the first 4-8 hours. Drink two ounces a day for the next five days—two tablespoons in the morning and two tablespoons in the night. Apply topically two to three times a day to the tumor if it is visible. In addition, you may find an intestinal cleansing daily with milk thistle beneficial. For more acute problems, drink four ounces one day and sip it every hour the next day.

If cancer runs in the immediate family, two tablespoons of a structured silver in the morning and evening can be used as a preventive method.

Maintaining a diet that is low in fat and sugar, and high in proteins, fiber, fruits and vegetables will also help. In addition, you want to get at least eight hours of sleep a night. You'll also want to take supplements that have immune-enhancing capabilities. You want to exercise if possible on a daily basis. I'm not talking strenuous, but just a walking type of exercise to make sure your circulation is good and your body's immune function is properly working in concert with your lymph system. You want to neutralize toxins in your air and water using proper filtration in your home. You want to cleanse the intestines and your blood. You cleanse the intestines with an intestinal cleanse, you cleanse your liver by using milk thistle on a daily basis in a supplement form, then you cleanse the bloodstream by taking a large amount of antioxidants. And you want to eliminate as much stress as you possibly can.

Antiviral

Viruses cause many diseases that we don't have pharmaceutical drugs to cure. For this reason, the human race is at a high risk for virus activity. We have viruses that are being treated incorrectly with antibiotics. Antibiotics do nothing to destroy or cure viral infections. Structured silver is very powerful and functions against both reverse transcriptase and DNA polymerase viruses, interfering with their replication process.

By drinking two tablespoons of structured silver in the morning and night, you can potentially defeat an existing viral infection. Inhaling a nebulized form of silver works best for a viral infection in the lungs or sinuses. Drops can also be placed in your ears, eyes, nose, or throat twice a day.

To prevent a cold or flu, drink one teaspoon twice a day. If you are exposed to a lot of coughing and sneezing, the dose can be doubled. Immune-stimulating herbs are also beneficial.

Viruses are very difficult to kill using pharmaceutical medicines because antibiotics do not kill viruses. The best way to destroy a virus is to put structured silver liquid, gel or mist in contact with the virus for 6 minutes. Many viruses infect young children and never fully leave the body. They stay dormant until the immune system becomes weak or stressed and then up comes the virus years later.

A person with AIDS has to deal with a virus that doesn't ever leave. Several AIDS patients have used silver liquid orally. They have swallowed one ounce or the liquid silver twice a day and found significant reduction of symptoms in three months, with some reporting to their doctors that all symptoms were gone. At this point they continue to use half the dose for maintenance. These patients used the treatments their doctors gave them and took the silver one hour staggered with their drugs. It should be noted that many AIDS patients have used the silver liquid in a dose as large as 4 ounces a day, and many have used this silver alone without any prescription medications and the results were similar to those patients using the prescription and silver protocols.

Antibiotic Alternative

According to Dr. Rustum Roy (Penn State University) silver is more broad-spectrum than anything found in the drug world or nature. This means structured silver kills more than just a tiny segment of bacteria, like antibiotics do. Structured silver kills all the bacteria except the healthy (probiotic) bacteria. This can happen because the healthy flora (lactobacillus) secretes a protective layer or lactobacillus around itself to protect against the acidic stomach acids. This protective layer prohibits the silver from rupturing the cell membrane because it cannot penetrate through the lactobacillus outer coating. This is demonstrated when a person takes antibiotics, and the action of the drugs kill the healthy flora, resulting in diarrhea. This is not seen when a person takes a quadruple dose of structured silver. In fact I have swallowed 8 ounces at one time (a 48 times normal dose) and never produced diarrhea. Remember it is the structured silver that improves antibiotic function and makes antibiotics up to ten times stronger when taken with structured silver. It should be noted that a person taking silver daily (1 teaspoon 1-3 times a day) should destroy bacterium, viruses and yeast that cause the majority of illnesses, so you may never need to take an antibiotic again. According to a study performed by Nelson Labs, structured silver was found to completely kill all tested bacteria and cause no resistance. This is important because it proves that structured silver is not going to cause the bacteria to get stronger or have the problems that plague antibiotic drugs.

Appetite Suppressant

Many people who suffer from overeating say they just can't seem to satisfy their appetite. Food cravings can be increased by an intestinal yeast growth that puts neurotoxins into the bloodstream. This creates damage everywhere the blood circulates, including the brain. Yeast is fed by sugar, and causes the body to crave more sugar.

Structured silver will not directly control your appetite nor suppress it. However, if you have a yeast infection, silver can kill the yeast in your intestines, decreasing neurotoxins and food cravings.

Structured silver should be considered for any dietary plan. One teaspoon twice a day will help maintain wellness. A digestive cleanse will also be beneficial.

Arthritis

Arthritis is characterized by painful swelling and inflammation in the joints. This can happen when uric acid is not excreted from the body quickly enough and is deposited in the joints of the toe, ankle, or knee. It can recrystallize, creating the same effect has having sand crystals between your joints. This damages the joint directly, causing inflammation around the joint and inflaming muscles, tendons, and cartilage.

By drinking two teaspoons twice a day, or as needed, structured silver can help reduce pain and inflammation. Silver gel can also be applied topically to the joint if it is hot or red. Glucosamine, chondroitin sulfate, and essential fatty acids may also be used.

Asthma

Asthma occurs when the bronchioles—the breathing tubes of the body and lungs—become inflamed and swell shut, preventing the body from drawing oxygen into the lungs. This results in choking, coughing, and heavy mucus production that can clog the breathing tubes to the point of asphyxiation.

To reduce inflammation, inhale structured silver from a nebulizer for 15 minutes in the morning and at a night. One teaspoon of silver liquid should also be taken twice a day. The gel can be placed inside the nostrils as a lubricant to help prevent against triggers for an asthma attack. Probiotics can also help reduce inflammation that originates from the digestive tract.

Athlete's Foot

Athlete's foot is basically a fungal infection on the skin. It occurs when we put our feet in shoes and keep them in a warm, moist area where fungus can grow. The first step to prevention is to wear clean shoes and reduce the amount of time that your foot stays in a moist sock.

Structured silver can be sprayed into your socks or directly on the foot. Structured silver gel is an even better option in this situation. It can be applied between the toes to kill any yeast growth. You can also spray silver into your shoes to kill any bacteria. In addition to athlete's foot, fungus can get underneath your toenails. By soaking your feet for 30 minutes every other day in a structured silver bath, you will kill the toenail fungus and the athlete's foot. The fungus will return if you continue to wear shoes or socks that are housing bacteria or fungus.

By killing the bacteria and yeast, structured silver will also remove the odor associated with athlete's foot.

Autism

We don't know all the causes of autism. It affects people of all ages, but seems to develop early in life. Autism has also been associated with some vaccinations and

A professional athlete developed foot and toenail fungus during his many years playing basketball. His feet were rough and scaly and toenails had become deformed and dark where the fungus existed. His feet stunk and were an embarrassment and public nuisance to be around in the showers and locker room.

He used a finger cot (a small latex balloon resembling a condom but for fingers), which he filled half full with silver gel and stretched it over his infected toes. After every shower he would scrub his feet and apply the silver gel to his feet and toes, then stretch the silver-filled cots over his infected toes. The gel was forced under his toenails where he kept it in the cot for at least 6 minutes and as long as 30 minutes nightly. He noticed improvements within three days and improvement continued until the toenails grew out (6 months later). His feet improved in three days and continued to improve as long as he soaked them in water, then scrubbed them and applied gel every day. Missing one day wasn't detrimental but missing two or more days stopped the progress.

inoculations. Antioxidants will help improve an autistic situation.

One class of autistic children who drank one teaspoon of a structured silver morning and night showed improved behavior, were less irritated and agitated, learned better, and asked more intellectual questions. Though it did not cure their autism, it did improve their symptoms. Children weighing more than 75 pounds should take two teaspoons morning and night. Probiotics, arginine supplementation, and phosphatitle serine may also help.

Backache

Structured silver has been shown to improve backaches associated with or caused by irritations on the skin or muscle tension. Applying the gel one to four times a day can help reduce pain and inflammation. Structured silver will not help a backache caused by bone problems.

Bacteria

Bacteria are single-cell organisms that actually grow within or outside your body. Left uninhibited, bacteria can cause disease or death. Many of today's health problems result from bacteria. Pneumonia, one of the leading causes of death in America, comes from bacteria inside of the lungs.

Structured silver will destroy bacteria in approximately six minutes. You will feel the effects within the first two hours of use and the benefits will continue as long as you use the product. Structured silver should also be combined with vitamins, minerals, essential fatty acids, amino acids, and antioxidants.

Bad Breath

Bacteria residing in the mouth and gums or between the teeth usually cause bad breath. Using a silver rinse can destroy these bacteria. By rinsing the mouth for six minutes in the morning and at night, you will get rid of the bad breath.

Bad breath can also be caused by strep throat or a staph infection. In these cases, bacteria destroy the healthy tissue, causing red blisters and white pus to form in the back of throat. The odor comes as a result of the degenerating tissue. Structured silver is the fastest way to remedy the problem.

Spraying structured silver into the nose four times a day can treat odor caused by a sinus infection.

Many people suffer bad breath because there is bacteria or yeast growing in their mouth between teeth, on the tongue, or from sinus drainage. The cause of offensive smelling breath in one person was from the gums being infected and continuously bleeding. The cause of her bleeding gums was from the bacteria that had been growing for years in between her teeth and in her gums.

The dentist diagnosed this as pyorrhea (gum disease) and referred her to a cardiologist because the bacterium in her gums was getting into her blood during bleeding. Every time she brushed her teeth her gums would bleed for a few minutes and the bacteria would enter her bleeding gums where her doctor diagnosed heart disease. In response to her doctor's prescription for heart-related conditions, she would rinse her mouth with silver liquid twice a day. This killed the bacterium that was causing her bad breath and because she swallowed the silver liquid after rinsing, she was able to help destroy the bacterial infection afflicting the arteries of her heart. After three months she had no bad breath, no bacteria in her mouth and her heart medication was reduced.

Bedsores

When a bed does not have proper balance, pressure points can form. Irritation or rashes on the skin then lead to open wounds. To treat bedsores, get a good bed with a neutral balance. Do not use too much laundry detergent on bedding and sheets.

Structured silver gel can be applied directly to the bedsore one to four times a day. The gel should be kept in place with a sterile bandage. You can expect improvement to begin very quickly after the gel is introduced to a wound. Improvement in diabetics may take two to three times longer because of circulation problems.

Black Mold

Black mold is a fungus or yeast that grows in wet areas of the home like showers or walls. The mold will release spores into the air. If these spores reach your lungs, they will produce asthma- and chronic-fatigue-like symptoms.

To remove the mold, spray liquid structured silver on it and let it stand for 10 minutes before wiping it off. This will destroy the mold and likely prevent it from re-growing.

Bladder Infection

Urine remains in the bladder for about six hours before it is drained. If bacteria get into the bladder, it will duplicate every 20 minutes—a bladder infection can become serious very quickly. The infection will degrade the lining of the bladder and possibly travel up the tubes from the bladder to the kidneys, causing a kidney infection.

To treat a bladder infection, two tablespoons of silver liquid should be taken hourly for the first two days. For the next two weeks, take two tablespoons twice a day. You may expect to destroy the bladder infection within the first 12 to 24 hours.

Structured silver liquid can be taken with cranberry juice or juniper berries.

Body Odor

Since bacteria causes most body odor, structured silver can help control the production of odor. Spray or apply silver to the affected area and drink one teaspoon twice daily. This can also help with bad breath.

Blood Cleanser

Bacteria, viruses, yeast, parasites, and other toxins can get inside our blood. Structured silver is one of the best tools for blood cleansing. It will enter a single red blood cell and cleanse at the cellular level.

I was on a trip to Asia when I got a bladder infection. In about 24 hours my bladder infection progressed from burning when I urinated, to passing blood.

I went to the doctor to find out what type of bacterial infection I had, so I could know what kind of antibiotics to take. Twelve hours before my doctor's appointment I started taking structured silver liquid. I drank one ounce each hour for four hours and then went to a two teaspoons twice a day maintenance dose.

By the time I got to the doctor and gave a urine sample, I was bacteria-free. There was a hint of blood, but no bacteria. The doctors were absolutely baffled by how such a severe bladder infection could be cleared up so quickly. The answer was simple. I took a large amount of structured silver liquid and it destroyed the bacteria in my bladder. The doctor said I didn't even need to take antibiotics.

If you have bleeding or serious pain during urination, it is important to see a doctor.

For acute blood cleansing, take one ounce every hour for four hours. For some serious conditions, you will need to take one four ounce bottle every day for the first three days, followed by a maintenance dose of two tablespoons twice a day.

To cleanse your blood each day, take one to two teaspoons, one to three times a day. Vitamin E in soft gel form may also help.

Boils

Boils occur when bacteria or viruses get under the skin and duplicate, destroying the healthy tissue. The duplication produces a pustule, which is similar to cystic acne, only it doesn't need a hair follicle or sebaceous gland to get down into the skin. Boils can be caused by simple irritations such as the rubbing of a belt on the skin or agitation on the side of a foot.

Applying a silver gel topically one to four times a day can treat a boil. In some cases, you may want to cover the boil with a bandage. In addition, you will want to drink two teaspoons of structured silver liquid twice a day.

As soon as the liquid and the gel come in contact with the bacteria, the boil growth will stop. Within about two hours you'll feel inflammation reduction. You will see improvement of the boil within four hours.

Bones

Bones can have a number of problems—breaks, infections, stoppage in the production of bone marrow and red blood cells—and pain is almost always associated with these problems. Structured silver liquid taken on a daily basis can help reduce the bacteria, virus, and mold within the system, thus reducing the impact on the bones.

Structured silver can help reduce the infection rate associated with broken bones or compound fractures, allowing the immune system to repair the bone much quicker. Calcium and magnesium may also be used.

Bowels

Bowels can have a lot of problems—from constipation and colitis to infections, diarrhea, and yeast infections. Taken regularly, structured silver liquid can help destroy the bacteria and yeast that cause many of these problems.

While regular cleanses are very efficient at removing constipation and toxins, often they do not remedy the cause of the problem, which may be yeast or bacteria.

Structured silver can help destroy the cause of the problem. You should expect to see benefits within the first two days.

Brain Cleansing

It is very difficult to get cleansing agents across the blood/brain barrier, but there are cases where the brain needs cleansing. The first step is to take white refined sugar out of your diet. The second step is to inhale silver liquid from a nebulizer. This allows the silver to travel through the nasal passages and lungs into the brain quicker and easier than through the bloodstream. Inhale the mist 30 minutes a day and take two teaspoons of structured silver twice a day.

Breast Cancer

High levels of bad estrogens, toxins, radiation, and many other problems can cause breast cancer. It has been estimated that as many as 60 percent of all cancers have a bacterial cause.

Drinking structured silver in the following doses can help prevent bacteria from causing cancer: Four ounces day one and four more ounces day two, sipping it every hour; two ounces a day for the next five days.

Drink two tablespoons in the morning and two tablespoons at night for maintenance. You can apply the structured silver gel topically two to three times a day as well. Antioxidants will also be beneficial.

Radiation treatment can burn the skin. Applying a silver gel in combination with aloe to the affected area will help prevent cellular damage and reduce pain.

Bronchitis

Bronchitis can be bacterial or a virus that causes the inflammation of the bronchioles—the tubes that the pass air from the throat down into the lungs.

Bronchitis results in excess mucus production, clogged lungs, and coughing.

Bronchitis can be cleared up by drinking two teaspoons of structured silver two to four times a day, inhaling silver from a nebulizer 15 minutes twice a day, and by using an intra-nasal spray twice a day for congestion.

For those living, working, or traveling with someone with bronchitis, spray structured silver into the nose for prevention. The gel can also be applied to the inside of the nostrils. Immune-stimulating herbs and coenzyme Q10 will also help. A cellular cleanse will prevent toxins and bacteria and viruses from gaining access blood stream.

A few years back, I injured myself very badly. I broke the orbital bone over my eye and had to have 15 stitches. This resulted in the biggest black eye I had ever seen. My eye was swollen shut. The bruise was dark purple because veins had ruptured around my eye.

I applied structured silver gel four times a day and took two teaspoons of structured silver liquid twice a day. The attending physician, Colonel Molof, a top military doctor, said it healed three times faster than any comparable wound he'd ever seen.

The injury healed so quickly because the gel killed all of the bacteria and mold that may have been impeding the immune system from doing its job. Structured silver also reduces inflammation at the same time.

Bruises

Bruises occur when a blood vessel is ruptured and blood pools in the tissue around it. Bruising often results from impact, but can also be caused by bacterial or viral infections. It can also occur when blood doesn't clot well.

Structured silver helps remove the blood from the tissue, improving the bruise. Simply soak a sterile bandage in liquid silver and place it on the bruise. Structured silver gel can also be applied to the wound one to four times a day.

Bug Bites

When a bug bites you or you are stung by a bee, toxins are introduced into your system. Structured silver helps by reducing inflammation and pain and improves wound healing. A bandage soaked in structured silver can be applied directly to the bite. Drinking one ounce of structured silver liquid twice a day for two days will also lessen tissue damage and improve toxin excretion. You can expect faster improvement and less inflammation.

Burns

Burns occur from the sun, radiation, x-rays, fire, heat, and from other chemicals in our environment. Structured silver is at its very best when it's used to treat a burn. It reduces pain and inflammation and improves wound healing. Structured silver liquid can be sprayed on the burn or used to soak the burn, and the gel can be applied to the wound where a significant reduction in pain, inflammation and tissue damage will be visible in the first hour.

Often burn wounds are so painful that you will want to spray on structured silver liquid or use a silver gel that has an aloe mixed with it to help with the pain. The gel will stay on the wound for a long period of time. The liquid will get into the wound very quickly, but needs to be reapplied every few hours. Drink one ounce of structured silver liquid twice a day until the burn is gone.

I know a fair-skinned young man who went to the beach and got very badly sunburned. We took a photo of his face and then applied the silver gel to just one half of his face. This would allow him to see the effects of silver as compared to his untreated skin.

The gel side did not ever blister, the redness faded quickly and the pain was resolved in minutes. The untreated side of his face blistered and peeled, taking about a week and a half to heal. It was painful, red, and irritated. Structured silver works on the worst of burns.

An 80-year-old woman suffered third-degree burns when a pot of coffee fell in her lap. The wounds from her thigh to her knee were so deep she could not even receive a skin graft. Her doctors were considering surgery to deal with the burn.

Instead they took a chance and tried structured silver gel. The gel was applied twice a day. In 66 days she was absolutely healed. The wounds had become absolutely scar-free, with just a few lines showing where she had been burned. Equally important, she did not have to take pain-killing drugs throughout the process.

Cancer

While silver has proven promising against many health conditions, those who have cancer or who may suspect they have cancer should always consult a physician before pursuing any course of treatment.

Cancer is always caused by a multiplicity of factors. Toxins, poisons, and pesticides have all been proven to cause cancers. Bacteria are one of the greatest causes of cancer because they can neutralize your immune system, allowing damage inside the cell on the DNA level. It is estimated that up to 60 percent of all cancers have a root in bacterial causes.

Structured silver is a broad-spectrum preventive agent. It destroys bacteria in as little as 15 seconds and kills the viruses and mold that may also cause cancer.

Those suffering from cancer should drink four ounces of structured silver on day one and four ounces on day two, sipping it every hour. Drink two ounces a day for the next five days; take two tablespoons twice a day thereafter as a maintenance dose.

Sinus, mouth, throat, or lung cancer patients may want to use an inhaled form of liquid structured silver. One ounce can be inhaled from a nebulizer 30 minutes a day. This allows the structured silver to come in deep contact with the lungs, bronchioles, and sinuses. This approach should be combined with oral structured silver use.

There is also a very experimental method for IV usage. About 3,000 cases have used structured silver intravenously, with no reported toxicity problems. An IV can be made utilizing 250 CCs of structured silver liquid at 10 parts per million. Mix one to one with a D5W mixture hung in a bag and dripped for one hour, given every other day for 10 total doses.

It should be noted that saline solution cannot be used because the salts in the saline inactivate the structured silver. This is a very important formulation and can be adjusted in any parts per million of the structured silver. Using the mathematical proportion of 250 CCs, you can use any part per million that you need to begin with.

When you put structured silver liquid directly in the veins it can begin killing even the most serious bacteria in 15 seconds. Noticeable improvements have been show to occur within the first two days. It has shown to be promising against viral infections like hepatitis, against cancer, and even against Epstein-Barr and the AIDS virus. Milk thistle can be used as a liver and intestinal cleanse. Drinking antioxidants daily will help cleanse the blood as well.

Silver and Cellular Abnormalities: According to the Journal of Chem. Medicinal Chem. (Nov. 2007), beams of ultraviolet light can be used to destroy tumors and cancers. Special molecules are injected into the bloodstream and then activated by a beam of ultraviolet light. It only takes a few minutes of light beam therapy to actively attack the cancer cells. The top research scientist, Colin Self, stated: "I would describe this development as the equivalent of ultra-specific magic bullets." This breakthrough in cancer treatment is significant to structured silver because, according to Penn State University Professor Roy, structured silver has been published to resonate at a frequency of 910 terahertz, which falls in the same category of ultraviolet light frequency as the anti-tumor lights (Curr. Science Invest, 2007).

It has been shown that infectious agents are associated with causing solid tumors (Kaposi's sarcoma), blood-based cancers (Leukemia) and other forms of cancers such as cervical cancer, which is caused by the Human Papilloma Virus(46). As you can see, bacteria, viruses, mold and other infectious agents have been reported to cause cancers. Taken daily, structured silver can prevent cellular bacteria, viruses, and mold so that the single-cell abnormalities never go beyond a single cell.

This is important because once diagnosed, doctors often prescribe chemotherapy or radiation that can cause immune suppression. This suppression of normal immune function allows for multiple pathogens to seed or spread. In this situation structured silver may have the potential to play a dual role: destroy the infectious agent that causes the cancer and/or destroy the pathogenic load arising from the immunocompromised patients.

Doctor Rentz[47] reports that the following cancer-associated infections are susceptible to structured silver treatment: HIV[48], Kaposi's sarcoma[49], Epstein Barr Virus[50], Respiratory syncytial virus[51], Influenza, Parainfluenza, Fungemia[52], Rotavirus[53] Cytomegalovirus[54], and streptococcus pneumoniae.[55]

Published cancer results include: "We studied malignant fibrosarcoma cells (cancerous fibro-blasts) and found that electrically injected silver suspended their runaway mitosis".[56] "Women with breast cancer (confirmed by biopsies), each received a single dose of a structured silver at a concentration of 10 ppm. The 30 subjects were re-tested by biopsy at day 19 post injection, resulting in 100% normal tissue".[57]

Canker Sores

Canker sores have a myriad of causes. Too much acid in the mouth is the number-one cause. The tissue in the mouth gets destroyed by stomach acid, too many sugars, and bacterial or viral infections.

A pH-balanced structured silver can help improve the issues quickly. Hold one ounce of pH-balanced structured silver liquid in your mouth for six minutes and then drink it. Repeat this process twice a day. Silver gel can also be applied topically to the wound.

If the canker sore is a result of the herpes virus, the sooner you get the gel on the wound, the sooner you can stop the virus from replicating and getting worse. You can expect the wound to improve twice as fast with structured silver gel applied to the canker sore than if it were to run its course normally.

Candida (see Yeast)

Cardiovascular Disease (Heart Disease)

Cardiovascular disease affects the heart, veins, arteries, and the circulation of blood and nutrients throughout the body. It is estimated that as much as 80 percent of all cardiovascular disease has its origin as a bacterial infection that originates in the mouth.

Cardiovascular disease can come from a bacterial infection like strep throat or a staph infection. By rinsing the mouth with structured silver liquid, you can kill the bacteria in the gums that lead to cardiovascular disease. This will also kill the bacteria that cause gum disease and bad breath.

Carpal Tunnel Syndrome

Carpal tunnel syndrome is characterized by painful swelling and inflammation in the joints. By drinking two teaspoons twice a day, or as needed, structured silver can help reduce pain and inflammation. Structured silver gel can be applied topically to the joint if it is hot or red. Glucosamine, chondroitin sulfate, and essential fatty acids may also be used.

Cataracts

Cataracts cloud your vision, distort your view, and make it difficult to read and focus. Fortunately, the condition can be prevented and improved. Apply two or three drops of liquid structured silver directly in the eyes one to four times a day and drink two teaspoons twice a day for one week, or until the problem is remedied. Other products that can help include bilberry eyebright, lutein, and antioxidants.

You may expect to have an improvement in your eyesight very quickly, especially if you have very dry eyes or a bacterial or viral infection. Cataracts that are very progressed are difficult to reverse, but the surface of the eye and the clarity of lens can be improved by using structured silver topically.

Cavities

Teeth are susceptible to cavities. Though the enamel is very hard, sugar and bacteria have the ability to eat away the enamel and cause cavities.

Rinsing your mouth with a structured silver regularly will kill cavity-causing bacteria. Rinse your mouth for six minutes with one ounce of liquid silver two times a day. Then swallow two teaspoons to benefit your entire body. Coenzyme Q10 will also help improve gum health.

I was on a trip with a man in his 30s. He started experiencing a lot of pain in a tooth and his gum line. The next day the mouth was more painful and it was very sensitive to water. It looked like he was starting to develop a cavity and an abscess was developing under his gum.

He took a finger full of structured silver gel, placed it on his gums and rubbed it in. He also rinsed his mouth with structured silver liquid for six minutes. Before he had even finished, the pain was reduced significantly. He did not have to suffer for the next few days until he could get to a dentist. The abscess also reduced in size.

In addition to brushing your teeth daily, I recommend brushing with structured silver gel once or twice a week. I also recommend a five-minute mouth rinse with a liquid once a week.

Chafing

Chafing occurs when skin rubs against skin or when another piece of clothing rubs against skin. The skin becomes reddened, a rash forms, and bleeding may occur. When applied to affected areas, structured silver gel will speed improvement and reduce pain.

A group of motorcyclists came in to see me after a long day of riding on the sand dunes. They all had chafed areas from where their bottoms and their inner thighs had rubbed against their seats and gas tanks all day. Sand had gotten in their pants and chafed them to the point that the skin was red and nearly bleeding.

They applied structured silver gel to these areas. Within five minutes, their pain was relieved and within two hours the redness was gone. By the next morning most of them had no problems at all. One rider had some scabbing, but it was pain-free and there was no inflammation.

Children

Structured silver is safe for use with children. Children require a smaller dose of liquid structured silver than adults. A 50-pound child, for instance, would take one-third the dosage of a 150-pound adult. Children will utilize the gel much more frequently, however, because they have poorer hygiene habits.

Silver gel can be given to children one to four times a day, and they can drink structured silver liquid once or twice a day. For prevention, I recommend children take one-half teaspoon once or twice a day. This general dosage may be doubled during times of illness.

Cholesterol

Cholesterol is found among the fats in the arteries and veins. If too much fat accumulates, the blood can thicken and the fat can stick anywhere it is circulated. The liver is responsible for the fat levels in your blood and arteries. If the liver is not working optimally, enzymes are not produced correctly, fats are overproduced, and the liver gets clogged with cholesterol. The liver is then unable to detoxify the body and cholesterol levels continue to increase.

Using a structured silver does not directly reduce cholesterol. However, by combining it with a healthy diet, exercise, a reduction in fats, and plenty of exercise and water, it can help the liver function properly and keep cholesterol at a normal range. Take one teaspoon of structured silver morning and night. I would also recommend a liver cleanse with milk thistle.

Chicken Pox

Because chicken pox is a virus, structured silver can be very beneficial in neutralizing the problem. It can also help with the associated blistering and scarring. By applying the gel within four hours of the first outbreak, structured silver can help reduce the impact to the skin. Often the blisters will not completely arise and scarring will be lessened.

If you already have blisters, applying the gel topically one to four times a day will help conditions improve quickly. In addition, you should drink two teaspoons of structured silver twice a day. Chicken pox can return years later in the form of shingles. This dosage will also help with shingles.

Chlamydia

Chlamydia is a bacterium that is transferred by sexual contact. It destroys the tissues inside the vagina and can reoccur when the immune system is depressed. It is informally referred to as "clap."

Bacteria inside the vagina and surrounding area cause Chlamydia. The symptoms of Chlamydia include pain, inflammation, rash and tissue damage.

- Drink two teaspoons of structured silver liquid twice a day for prevention.
- Use a silver gel as a personal lubricant on the male and female genitals, prior to sex. The gel is water-soluble and lubricates just like KY Jelly. Structured silver gel has potential to act against sexually transmitted diseases like gonorrhea, syphilis, AIDS, Herpes simplex and Chlamydia. You can also put gel on a condom to lubricate and destroy bacteria, viruses, and yeast that may be transferred during intercourse.

Chronic Fatigue Syndrome

Chronic fatigue syndrome has a number of different causes—viral, bacterial, hormonal, or parasitic. Important identifying factors include muscle and joint aches, stiffness, and fatigue. It can also affect hearing and eyesight.

Two tablespoons of structured silver can be taken two or three times a day for relief. Gel can be applied or sprayed on sore muscles once or twice a day as needed for aches and pains. Structured silver liquid drops can be used in the eyes and ears as well.

Many people suffering from Epstein bar virus or mononucleosis have taken structured silver to help restore their energy. Additional products to help with chronic fatigue are coenzyme Q10 and free-form amino acids.

Circulation (See also Cardiovascular Disease)

Circulation can be improved simply by taking the bacteria, viruses, and yeast out of the system. In addition to drinking two teaspoons of structured silver a day, use of vitamin E, dietary fiber, and antioxidant drinks can help.

Cleansing

Structured silver helps cleanse the organs of excretion (colon, bladder, kidneys, etc.) by killing the bacteria, viruses and yeast that infect them. Remember it takes 6 minutes for the structured silver to completely kill these pathogens. In a cleansing situation structured silver will kill about 80% of the pathogen in as little as 15 seconds but if you keep the liquid or gel in contact with the pathogen for 6 minutes you will destroy the pathogen completely in almost all cases. Most people will use structured silver liquid 2 teaspoons twice a day. Apply the gel as needed to affected areas.

Colds

Colds are a virus. A cold gets in your nose and your sinuses and starts to duplicate there, producing a lot of mucus. Many will experience postnasal drip—mucus dripping down the back of the sinuses into the throat—when they go to bed. The mucus contains a virus or bacteria. When it reaches the back of the throat, it causes swelling and inflammation and can even spread into the ears.

Taking one tablespoon of structured silver three times a day, and spraying intranasally four or five times a day, will help reduce congestion and inflammation. Mouth rinse, ear drops, eye drops, nose drops, and throat spray can all be used as well.

Colitis, Irritable Bowel Syndrome, and Diverticulitis

Colitis is an inflamed colon. Irritable bowel syndrome is characterized by irritated and swollen bowels, and alternating constipation and diarrhea. Diverticulitis results from overstretched intestines that collect toxins—the body starts absorbing the toxins that should be passing out of the body and the toxins can get into the bloodstream.

By taking two teaspoons twice a day, liquid silver can kill the yeast that causes these ailments. Herbs like cats claw, digestive enzymes, and acidophilus will also help.

Colon (See Enema)

Compress

Silver gel taken from a refrigerator and put on a sterile gauze bandage can be used as a compress for bruises and wounds. It can help bring down a fever and help compress sore or inflamed parts of the body. The cold temperature aids as a cold pack.

Congestion

Congestion—including nasal, lung, and upper respiratory—can stop you from breathing properly. Congestion leads to high production of mucus and can clog the nose, throat, sinuses, and lungs. If bacteria cause the congestion, it can last for months if the bacteria are not destroyed.

To remove congestion, spray structured silver into your nose one to four times a day and drink two teaspoons of the liquid twice a day. Inhaling silver 30 minutes a day in nebulized form can help lung congestion.

Congestion can create a poor sleep pattern and lead to decreased immune function. A hot, steamy shower will help you clean out your sinuses. Once the sinuses are clean, spray structured silver high into the nostrils using a nasal atomizer. Rinse your mouth with structured silver as well, swallowing the solution when finished.

Constipation

Constipation has many causes, but foremost is lack of water. Bacterial or viral infections can create distress in your intestinal walls and decrease ability to absorb the proper amounts of water. Structured silver can be of benefit when you drink one to two teaspoons twice a day. Acidophilus, fiber, and cleansing herbs will also help.

By keeping constipation at a minimum, you will keep toxins out of your bloodstream and neurotoxins out of your brain. You will cleanse all parts of your body and prevent the liver from becoming overloaded with detoxification work.

Conjunctivitis (Pink Eye)

Conjunctivitis results when bacteria build up on the surface of the eye. It can actually change the white of your eye, causing it to swell and turn pinkish red. If the inflammation is not reduced, the eyesight can be permanently damaged.

Structured silver can help when you apply two or three drops of liquid structured silver directly into the eyes one to four times a day. Structured silver gel can be placed directly into the eye where the gel will stay in place longer. Drink two teaspoons twice a day for one week or until the problem is remedied. This will usually remedy the problem within the first two to three days. Additional products that help are bilberry, eyebright, and lutein.

Crohn's Disease

Crohn's disease is an inflammation of irritable bowel syndrome. The main symptoms are abdominal pain, diarrhea (which may be bloody, though this may not be visible to the naked eye), constipation, vomiting, weight loss, or weight gain. Though it is an infection, it is not clear if it is caused by bacteria, a virus, a parasite, or all three. By drinking four ounces of liquid structured silver the first day and two teaspoons of structured silver per day thereafter, you can destroy all three potential causes of the symptoms. Crohn's disease is an autoimmune disease because the body attacks itself. For this reason silver is very good at destroying pathogens without inflaming the immune system.

In addition to structured silver liquid on a daily basis, you may want to consider adding acidophilus, cats claw, and coenzyme Q10.

Cuticles

For cuticle care, soak your fingers in structured silver liquid for 30 minutes or apply a silver gel with a moisturizing agent like aloe. For cracked, dry cuticles, cover the hands with rubber gloves after applying the silver gel to seal in moisture.

Cysts

Cysts are usually the result of bacteria that collects under the skin. It grows and produces puss or other kinds of toxins. Take two teaspoons of liquid structured silver twice a day and apply the gel topically four times a day.

Dandruff

Dandruff is usually caused by dry, flaky skin. It can also be aggravated by a fungal or a bacterial infection. Apply structured silver to the scalp, rub it in, and allow it to stand for 10 minutes. This will stop bacterial and fungal infection and keep the scalp moist, reducing flaking.

Dengue Fever

Dengue Fever is an acute febrile disease found in the tropics and Africa. It is caused by four closely related viruses. Structured silver can help when inhaled from a nebulizer 30 minutes a day and by drinking two teaspoons twice a day.

Unfortunately, Dengue fever can often get into parts of the body the silver has difficulty reaching. If this happens, increase the dosage to one teaspoon six times a day. If this doesn't work after two days, drink one full ounce and then return to the original dosage.

Depression

Depression can occur for a lot of different reasons, including biochemical and hormonal imbalances. A sedentary lifestyle can also lead to depression.

When a person has a depressed system, their chemistry needs to get back into balance. This isn't always easy. It requires a healthy diet and exercise. It has been found that people exercising 90 minutes a week over the course of eight weeks were able to control depression better than by taking antidepressant pharmaceutical drugs.

Bacterial and viral infections can have an effect on depression as well. Drinking one teaspoon of structured silver twice daily can keep these infections under control. St. John's Wort can help with mild to moderate depression and coenzyme Q10 can help with energy. A digestive parasite cleanse combined with structured silver can also improve depression by taking some of the toxins out of the intestinal system. Liquid structured silver can be taken one to two teaspoons one to three times a day.

Dermal Renewal

The dermis is a layer of the skin. The top layer of skin is basically dead. When we wash the skin the top layer flakes off. Deeper in the dermis, there is a continuous growth of new cells, producing new layers of healthy skin and tissues.

To help with dermal renewal, apply a structured silver gel to skin anywhere on the body and then cover it with a plastic wrap. This keeps the gel from evaporating and allows it to penetrate deeper dermal layers of the skin. In addition, drink one teaspoon of liquid structured silver twice a day.

Detox Bath

Sometimes people want to rinse everything off their body—bacteria, viruses, mold, chemical substances, pollution, etc. To create a detox bath, fill your bathtub with warm water, pour in four ounces of liquid structured silver, and bathe for 20 minutes. This will allow you to wash every orifice of your body and all of your skin. Apply structured silver gel to your body after you get out, while the skin is still moist.

Diabetes

Diabetes is a problem associated with the islets of Langerhans cells in the pancreas. When these islets cells don't function properly, insulin is not produced and blood sugar gets out of balance. Those with no function in the islet of Langerhans or total pancreatic failure have Type I diabetes. In Type II diabetes, the islets of Langerhans cells have partial or damaged function.

One way that damage to the pancreas can be caused is by bacterial and viral infections. Drinking two teaspoons of structured silver twice daily can help fight these types of infections. Amino acids, coenzyme Q10, exercise, and healthy diet (with little to no refined sugars) will be beneficial.

Structured silver does not cure diabetes; it helps prevent damage to the pancreas before diabetes sets in. Structured silver gel can improve diabetic ulcers and wounds and is especially beneficial for foot wounds, venous stasis, ulcers, hemorrhoids, and varicose veins. Use the structured silver gel one to four times a day to keep these ulcers moist so they can improve more quickly.

Diarrhea and Dysentery

Diarrhea can be caused by a bacteria or virus. Dysentery is a bacterial infection. By taking a teaspoon of structured silver in the morning and at night, you can prevent these infections.

If you already have diarrhea or dysentery, you should swallow two teaspoons every hour for the first eight hours. The structured silver will help in as little as four hours. Complete improvement may take up to two days. Acidophilus can also be used.

I experienced food poisoning and diarrhea after eating airplane food. I drank one ounce of structured silver every hour for the first two hours. My diarrhea stopped and I didn't have any further serious problems. This relief was very important because I had to continue traveling on the plane.

Diaper Rash

When babies wear diapers their skin can be in contact with urine for long periods of time. This warm, moist area of the skin will allow bacteria and fungus to grow very quickly. The skin becomes red and can even crack or bleed. By applying silver gel to the diaper rash you will be able to kill the cause of the diaper rash in the first two hours. The redness and pain can be remedied in as little as five minutes in mild cases.

To prevent diaper rash, you can spray a thin layer of structured silver on the inside of the diaper and then allow it to stand for about two minutes. This approach can also be used in children's socks to prevent athlete's foot.

Digestive System

Some common digestive system problems include excessive gas, diarrhea, yeast infections, or stabbing pains associated with a bacterial infection or food poisoning. Structured silver liquid can help with each of these conditions. Drink two teaspoons every hour for about eight hours to help your digestive system. For daily prevention, drink one teaspoon twice a day.

Diverticulitis and Diverticulosis (See Colitis)

Babies develop diaper rash due to bacteria or yeast being placed in a warm moist environment against the baby's skin. The rash is very red, and painful and baby and parent get little or no sleep until remedied. Physicians often prescribe antibiotic ointments and even cortisone for the residual rash sometimes. This mom chose to use silver gel applied directly to the afflicted area three times a day and after two hours the redness was gone the baby had fallen asleep and the problem totally remedied within 4 hours. I have seen similar results hundreds of times and the most common way to prevent diaper rash is to apply silver gel to the baby's bottom every time it gets wet and let the gel dry in the open air for one minute before applying the diaper. It has been seen that silver gel can function as a painkiller in as little as 5-7 minutes for diaper rash.

Dry Skin

Dry skin occurs because we don't have enough fluids, oils, or essential fatty acids in our skin. It can also be caused by a bacterial infection, lack of exercise, or poor diet. Dry skin can lead to cracking, which allows infections to get into your system.

Structured silver liquid and gel in combination with aloe can be used to protect dry skin from infections. It should be applied to the dry skin one to four times a day. Silver liquid can be taken one teaspoon twice a day. Aloe vera, amino acids, vitamin E or flax oil supplements can also be used.

Ear Drops (See Ear Infections)

Ear Infections

Ear infections are a serious problem. In fact, Centers for Disease Control has requested that physicians no longer prescribe antibiotics for ear infections. The antibiotics make the problem worse by making the bacteria more resistant. We now have bacteria that we can't kill with antibiotics.

An ear infection can be a result of bacteria that gets in the inner ear and duplicates itself, destroying healthy tissue along the way. This could possibly leave a person deaf.

These bacteria can be destroyed by structured silver liquid after just five minutes of contact. Use a dropper to place five drops into the ear canal, or fill it complexly, while the ear is pointed towards the roof. Keep the ear tilted up for 12 minutes. This will allow the structured silver liquid to get as far down behind the ear as possible. Repeat this process in each ear every 12 hours. You will also want to drink two teaspoons of liquid structured silver twice daily and take vitamin C.

Endometriosis

Endometriosis is a condition where endometrial tissue is present outside of the uterus, causing severe uterine and/or pelvic pain.

The main symptom of endometriosis is pain concentrated in the lower abdomen. It may localize to one side of the abdomen or radiate to the thighs and low back. There is usually painful menstruation (dysmenorrhea), with different types of pain depending on the person—sharp, throbbing, dull, nauseating, burning, or shooting pains. Endometriosis may be long- or short-term; it may precede menstruation by several days or accompany it, but it usually subsides as menstruation tapers off. Severe pain may coexist with excessively heavy blood loss. On rare occasions nausea, vomiting, diarrhea, headache, dizziness or disorientation may occur.

Prostaglandins are inflammatory compounds released during menstruation that cause the muscles of the uterus to contract. Sometimes, the uterus muscles constrict so much that the blood supply is compressed, reducing the delivery of blood to the sensitive tissues of the endometrium. The absence of blood flow to the endometrium causes pain and cramping as the tissues die from lack of blood. The uterus begins to contract in such a strong manner that the dead tissues are squeezed out of the uterus and through the cervix and vagina. This temporary oxygen deprivation in the uterus is responsible for the cramps and pain. Silver makes dramatic improvements in wound healing and pain management inside the uterus. It also reduces inflammation, which can help reduce the cause of this painful disease.

· Swallow two tsps of structured silver liquid twice a day for prevention and treatment.

- Apply structured silver gel topically to affected area 2-5 times a day for as long as needed. You can also apply the gel to a tampon and insert into the vagina for 90 minutes a day. In this way the gel will stay in contact with wounds in the vagina.
- You can also create a structured silver douche. Use three ounces of structured silver liquid and mix it with three ounces of distilled water. Pump the solution into the vaginal cavity and hold for ten minutes, then release. This should be done once a day, for five days, or until symptoms are gone.
- There are optional uses of structured silver. Pour four ounces of structured silver liquid into a full tub of warm water. Soak and relax, flushing the silver water into the vaginal cavity. Twenty-five minutes is average for a muscle relaxing vaginal flush in the tub.

Enema

If you choose to use the silver as an enema it is most commonly used after the colonic or enema is completed and then a rinsing dose of 60 ml of structured silver liquid can be pumped into the colon. The gel can be used on the rectum to help prevent contamination or treat hemorrhoids.

Energy

When a person feels short on energy, their metabolism is usually in some form of disarray—often times the liver is damaged. By taking two teaspoons twice a day, structured silver has the ability to help restore proper function to the liver. This will help the liver secrete correct amounts of enzymes, detoxifying the body and allowing for more energy.

Enhances Antibiotic Function

Dr. Rustum Roy published studies that demonstrate the synergy of structured silver with antibiotics. Structured silver makes some antibiotics ten times more effective at killing bacteria.

Antibiotics are rarely used for more than two weeks because they produce supergerms if utilized too long. Structured silver does not produce this bacterial mutation because it destroys all the bacteria, resulting in a product that can be used daily without producing supergerms.

Epidemics, Pandemics

We are always at risk for an epidemic breakout, whether it is bacterial, viral, or parasitic. We've been warned that an influenza epidemic could kill as much as half of our population. Bird flu is also a real concern.

Liquid structured silver is one of the best tools in the event of an epidemic outbreak. The gel is necessary because most contagious diseases are transferred by hand contact. Silver gel used on hands will help prevent as much as 70 percent of all contagious diseases.

At least one gallon of structured silver should be stored for each person in a home storage site. In addition to its anti-disease agent, it can help with water purification—four drops of structured silver will purify an eight ounce glass of water in less than two minutes.

To keep water safe for storage, pour approximately 32 ounces of structured silver liquid into a 55-gallon barrel of water, wait 10 minutes, and then seal it up. The water will stay safe for approximately four years.

Structured silver can also be used topically, orally, intravaginally, intranasally, or inhaled. In the event of an epidemic, you may need any or all of these methods.

Epilepsy and Seizures

Epilepsy and seizures can by caused from a myriad of different situations. If it is bacterial or viral, structured silver can help. To help with seizures, drink one teaspoon twice daily.

In addition to liquid silver, put silver gel on your hands twice a day to help prevent contagious diseases from being transferred from your hand to your own body. Probiotics, phosphatidyl serine, coenzyme Q10 and minerals, B-vitamins, and essential fatty acids can also help.

Epstein-Barr Virus

Epstein-Barr virus causes mononucleosis and chronic fatigue syndrome. Structured silver has the ability to destroy viruses. Drink four ounces for two days, sipping every hour. Drink two ounces a day for the next five days. For maintenance, drink two tablespoons in the morning and at night. Use topically as needed.

If you have a uterine yeast infection at the same time, you can use structured silver as a douche, holding it for twelve minutes before releasing. If you need the gel for sore muscles, apply it topically and recognize that acidophilus, vitamins, minerals, and essential fatty acids with coenzyme Q10 may help.

Eyes

There are many problems that can develop within the eyes, both bacterial and viral. Most of them come from the outside, except for a few circulatory problems.

Apply two or three drops of silver liquid directly into the eyes one to four times a day and drink two teaspoons twice a day for one week, or until the problem is remedied. On a long-term basis, one teaspoon twice a day will suffice.

If you kill the bacteria and viruses on the surface of the eye you will reduce redness, inflammation and itchiness. Hopefully the proper tearing will be restored and you will have an eye that has a chance to heal itself fully.

After using structured silver, you should expect visible and noticeable differences in the first hour, with substantial improvements within two hours. Lutein, blueberry, and antioxidants also help.

Eye Wash Device

The proper use of an eye wash device can be very effective at delivering structured silver liquid into the eye. When there is a foreign object in the eye, structured silver liquid can be delivered using a specialized eye cap. This is also beneficial when used for eye infections, trauma or chronic conditions. Five drops of structured silver liquid can be used 1 to 5 times a day.

Eye Lift

Eyes seem to sag just from the effects of gravity. Skin holds itself together because of elasticity, which comes from elastin and collagen. By using structured silver, the cells of your skin can start to pull together a little tighter, and a little faster. Take structured silver gel out of the refrigerator and apply while cold. The skin will tighten and firm for about two hours.

Face Lift

By applying refrigerated structured silver to your face, you will remove bacteria, viruses, and mold and see toning and tightening effects.

This also works on dark circles under the eyes, which are sometimes caused by toxins. Put a little gel under your eyes every morning and night and the silver will remove the dark color.

Facial Mask

Most facial masks only peel the dead skin cells off the surface of the face. Structured silver can actually remove the toxins.

I recommend a powdered clay mix with added structured silver. When the clay is applied to the skin in liquid form, the silver can remove bacteria and firm and tighten the skin. The clay will remove oils and detoxify the skin, destroying the causes of acne and blemishes. Supplement by drinking one teaspoon of structured silver liquid twice a day.

Facial Peel

Some people use a facial peel to get down to the new and youthful layers of skin. These peels use harsh chemicals, basically burning the skin at the very top layer of its cells. By applying silver gel after a facial peel you'll experience quick improvements, better color, less pain and damage. You'll also get longer results with better cellular structure. One teaspoon of liquid silver should also be taken daily.

Facial Treatment

Silver can be used as a facial treatment to help with regeneration of damaged cells, and wound management. It can also treat acne, infections, and premature aging. You will get the deepest structured silver penetration by washing the face with a mild soap, patting it dry, and then applying the gel to the skin while it is still moist. The gel can also be applied after steaming the face. This will open up the sweat glands and hair follicles and the gel will get deeper into the skin.

Applying the gel allows structured silver nanoparticles to prevent infections by destroying bacteria, viruses, mold, and improve wound healing at the same time. It will also help prevent premature aging at the cellular level. You should also drink one teaspoon of liquid structured silver twice a day.

If you have sensitive skin, you will find that liquid silver and gel reduce inflammation, swelling, puffiness, and allergies.

Family Use

Families can utilize silver in countless ways around the home. It can be used to clean the shower or sink, to neutralize odors, or to freshen laundry. It is most beneficial, however, when used as a preventive agent. For a healthier family, each member should drink at least one teaspoon of structured silver once or twice a day. If there is an illness in the family, spray down the refrigerator, doorknobs, and bathrooms and increase the dosage to two teaspoons twice daily.

In the event of an epidemic like influenza or bird flu, there should be one gallon of silver stored in the home for each member of the family.

Fatigue (see Chronic Fatigue Syndrome)

Fertility

Many women have a difficult time getting pregnant. Bacterial or viral infection could be the cause. Structured silver should be taken orally, one teaspoon a day, to kill any infection inhibiting the ability to become fertile. Two ounces of silver may also be used as a douche, held intravaginally for 12 minutes and then released.

Men will want to drink one teaspoon twice a day and use structured silver gel as a personal lubricant to ensure bacteria is not transferred to the woman during intercourse. Amino acids, essential fatty acids, and antioxidants will also help fertility.

Fevers

Bacteria, viruses, mold, foreign pathogens, and even sunburns cause fevers. To break a fever, drink one teaspoon every hour (up to eight hours) until the fever breaks. Structured silver gel can also be refrigerated and then applied topically to the forehead, temples, or anywhere else the fever is found.

If a fever does not break before it reaches 104° seek the care of a health care professional.

Fibromyalgia

Fibromyalgia is an autoimmune disorder with multiple symptoms. Though a single cause has not been identified, yeast seems to be a common factor. Yeast can leave the intestines and go into the brain. It can also be a neurotoxin, producing fermented fruits and vegetables in the intestines that can cause low-dose alcohol toxicity.

By cleansing yeast out of the system, most fibromyalgia patients can control some of their symptoms. Drinking two tablespoons of structured silver two or three times a day can destroy yeast. Gel or spray can be applied to sore muscles once or twice a day as needed for pain or aches. In addition to liver cleansing, vitamins, minerals, and freeform amino acids will all help with fibromyalgia.

Fingers (also see Toenail Fungus)

If you have sore or cracked fingers or cuticles—or a yeast infection under your fingernails or toenails—a structured silver soak can help. Soak your fingers in small dish of silver liquid for 15 minutes at a time. The gel does not penetrate as deeply, but will stay in place throughout the day.

Follicle Detox

Shaving the face or legs can results in damaged hair follicles. Silver gel can be used as a shaving gel to reduce bacteria, inflammation, swelling, and scarring.

Food Poisoning

Food poisoning typically includes symptoms such as nausea, vomiting, abdominal cramping, and diarrhea. It occurs suddenly (within 48 hours) after consuming a contaminated food or drink. It is usually caused by bacteria and viruses.

To fight food poisoning requires aggressive structured silver use, drinking about one ounce immediately, followed by two tablespoons every hour for the next eight hours. For prevention, drink one to three teaspoons a day. This can be especially helpful when traveling to a foreign country.

You can actually spray structured silver on food to kill the pathogens that cause food poisoning. After spraying, let it stand for two minutes before eating. Taking liquid structured silver can also kill E. coli and salmonella.

Foot Bath

You should drink two tablespoons of structured silver before using a therapeutic foot bath. These baths use electrolysis, sending a positive current through one end of an electrode and out through a negative electrode. Because silver is the best conductor of electricity, it will help in detoxifying the foot bath.

You can also create your own foot bath by placing structured silver in a bowl or tub, or by simply soaking washcloths and wrapping them around your feet.

Foot Odor

A very aggressive way to treat the feet is to soak them in warm water for 15 minutes. This will soften the dead skin on the surface, which can be scraped off with a loofah. Now the skin is ready and open for the gel to be applied to the entire foot. There are some sea salt scrubs that seem to help scrape the dead skin off with much more aggression. Silver kills the bacteria that causes odor and can be used to deodorize armpits, feet, breath and has been used for hunters to neutralize their odor while hunting.

Foot Treatment Pack

Silver gel and liquid can be very effective at killing fungus, yeast or bacteria that cause diseases of the foot. Specialized toe cots can be filled with silver gel and placed over the toe where the gel is pumped into and under the toenail. Slightly abrading (sanding) the toenail before applying the gel will allow better delivery of the gel.

· Before applying silver gel or liquid, first wash the foot and then remove the damaged, dead or diseased skin and nails. Do this by trimming the toenail, sanding the toenail and/or exfoliating the skin. Toes should be cotted twice a week until the toenail grows out healthy. Silver gel can be applied to the foot twice a day after washing for use against bacteria and fungus.

Flu

The flu is a viral infection that can be prevented if silver is taken daily. The person that wants to prevent the flu should take structured silver liquid two teaspoons twice a day and inhale one tablespoon from an inhaler or nebulizer 30 minutes a day. If you already have the flu, continuation of the same protocol is recommended.

For more detailed information about the flu and silver, check the Studies at the back of this book.

Gallbladder Disease

Gallbladder disease results from a breakdown in the digestive system. It can be very painful and can disrupt lives. Yeast and bacteria play a role in the disease. To fight these causes, drink two tablespoons of structured silver twice daily for two weeks. Reduce the dose to one tablespoon twice daily for two more weeks, and then maintain one teaspoon a day. Utilizing a proper gallbladder and digestive cleansing will also speed up recovery.

Gargle (See Mouth Wash)

Gastritis and Gas

Gas can be produced from yeast and sugar mixing with fruits and vegetables in your intestines. It can also be produced directly from certain fruits, vegetables, and bacteria. Most people think that gas is produced by eating beans. In reality, a bacterium on the surface of the bean produces gas.

Structured silver can help because it destroys a bacterium that causes gas. If you have a gas outbreak—including painful air pressure in the intestines—take two teaspoons

> *Structured silver is the most effective product I have ever worked with and is ranked number one by my patients. Not only is it the most effective, but it is the most researched technology on the market today."*
>
> *– Female gynecologist*

every hour for the first few hours.

In addition, you might want to try acidophilus and a digestive cleanse. Digestive enzymes can also be of assistance.

Genital Herpes

Genital herpes is a virus affecting the genital area. Applying silver gel topically can help the outbreak improve more quickly. It should be placed on the genitals as soon as the outbreak occurs. In addition, drink two teaspoons of structured silver liquid twice a day. Daily silver use will also help prevent future outbreaks.

Geriatric/Elderly Use

People over age 50 can use structured silver as recommended. They can also take up to four times the normal recommendations if they have a serious or chronic illnesses, depressed immunity, anemia, or are around a large quantity of germs. The gel and liquid can be used in any orifice of the body.

Gingivitis

Structured silver can be placed into the dental floss container and disinfect the floss that carves food off the tooth and gums. It also cuts into the gums and can cause infections, so pour two tablespoons of liquid structured silver into the dental floss container and use this disinfectant floss between your teeth.

Hand Disinfectant

Drink two teaspoons of structured silver twice a day, and apply silver gel to your hands one to four times a day, to help prevent problems associated with contagious diseases.

The application of silver gel replaces the role of alcohol- or petroleum-based hand sanitizers. Alcohol-based products dry out the skin and can cause cracking of the skin. Petroleum-based products leave a greasy feeling or flaking as the product dries. In contrast, structured silver gel can comfortably sanitize hands for four hours without staining or causing other undesirable effects.

Hand Restoration

As we age, our hands are exposed to sunlight, cleansing agents, and drying agents. The skin gets wrinkled and damaged. By drinking one teaspoon of liquid structured silver twice a day, the silver will enter the red blood cells and work from the inside of the capillary system. Applying structured silver gel one to four times a day can benefit the topical layers of the skin.

Hay Fever (see Allergies)

Headaches

Headaches can be caused by a number of different factors including bacteria, viruses, mold, allergens, and hormones. Because the brain does not contain pain receptors you cannot have a brain ache, but the veins and arteries that flow through your head can cause pressure and the circulatory system can feel pain.

By reducing the bacteria and viruses, structured silver can reduce the pain in the head. Drink two teaspoons twice a day and put gel on the temples twice daily. This will also kill the yeast, bacteria, and viruses that pass through the intestines into the bloodstream.

Healing Gel

In a study performed for the Singapore Department of Homeland Security, it was shown that structured silver liquid and gel improve wound healing by a factor of three times. This means wounds close three times faster than normal. There can be three times less bacteria in the wound and inflammation is reduced by three times. This means it can help reduce scarring, even those existing scars or stretch marks.

Structured silver can be used topically as a healing gel on sunburns, scratches, scrapes, bites, or chemical burns. Because structured silver passes through the body unchanged, it produces no harmful metabolites and will help the healing process wherever the circulatory and capillary systems take it.

Silver gel should be used a minimum of once a day as a preventive agent and up to 12 times a day, as needed, to keep a wound moist. Structured silver can be sprayed on, applied topically, or poured on as a liquid.

Hemorrhoids

Hemorrhoids are basically varicose veins at the rectum. These veins get irritated and swollen, causing a lot of pain. They get stretched out of shape and rupture with the passage of feces.

Structured silver can help improve varicose veins by applying topically to the affected area twice a day or after every bowel movement. The gel can be used as a lubricant to help the stool move smoothly. It can also help inflamed tissues improve quickly. In addition, drink one teaspoon of liquid structured silver morning and night. A stool softener is also recommended.

I know a body builder who works out every day. He's very strong and muscular and also had hemorrhoids. They had become so bad that the doctors wanted to do surgery to remedy the problem.

He decided to try silver. He applied the gel every day and after every bowel movement. He saw improvement the very first week. By two weeks, he was no longer waiting to have surgery. Now, a year and a half later, the hemorrhoids are completely healed.

Heart Disease (See Cardiovascular Disease)

Hepatitis

Hepatitis is an inflammation of the liver that destroys its function and can be caused by viruses or bacteria. It is very difficult to treat but structured silver can be used in high doses to be beneficial. Structured silver liquid can be swallowed 4 ounces a day for the first two weeks, and then swallowed two tablespoons twice a day for the next 3.5 months. This is a four-month attack on hepatitis. Gel can be used anywhere there might be contamination or transfer of germs.

Several successful subjects have used the drugs interferon and ribavirin at their lowest prescribed doses in combination with this protocol of structured silver. The liver numbers were reduced to near normal in one month and back to normal in two months and symptom-free in four months.

Herpes Virus

Herpes viruses can affect the skin or the nervous system. When a herpes virus infects the inside or outside of the vagina, blisters and pain result.

The symptoms of the Herpes virus typically include water blisters inside and outside the vagina. These can be extremely painful depending on the severity of the lesions.

- Structured silver liquid: Swallow two teaspoons of silver liquid twice a day for prevention and treatment. Also, apply the gel topically to affected area 2-5 times a day for as long as needed. Silver gel can also be applied to a tampon and inserted into vagina for 90 minutes a day so the gel can stay in contact with germs in the vagina.
- To create a silver douche, use three ounces of structured silver liquid mixed with three ounces of distilled water. Pump the solution into the vaginal cavity and hold for ten minutes, then release. This should be done once a day, for five days, or until symptoms are gone.
- Take at least 8 billion active culture probiotic daily. Reduce dietary sugar and carbohydrates. And take large quantities of antioxidants daily. This can help neutralize and clear free radicals produced by pathogens.

Structured silver can destroy the virus that causes infections in fewer than six minutes. This means the silver needs to stays in contact with the pathogen for at least six minutes. Most women feel noticeably better in one day and may return to normal in as little as two to five days.

High Blood Pressure

Hormones, blood or water volume, a change in biochemistry, a brain problem, or various other problems can cause high blood pressure. Structured silver can reduce high blood pressure by helping the liver function normally and produce proper enzymes and cholesterol. Structured silver can be taken in a liquid form, drinking two teaspoons twice a day. Dietary fiber should also be used.

Household Disinfectant

Structured silver can be used as a disinfectant by spraying it on household items—toys, dishes, phones, purses, bathtubs, sinks, doorknobs, and so forth. After spraying items, let the solution stand for 10 minutes before

A 55-year-old male with high blood pressure took two teaspoons of a structured silver water twice a week and rinsed it in his mouth (6 min) once a day to kill the bacteria in his mouth. In addition, he ate antioxidant-rich healthy chocolate. The high antioxidants from the dark chocolate work synergistically with structured silver to kill the cause of most heart disease in the mouth and arteries, while the antioxidants reduce arterial inflammation and help remove the circulatory pathogens killed by the silver. The two actions reduce high blood pressure.

wiping off. This will kill the bacteria throughout your home. Structured silver gel can also be used, offering four hours of disinfectant power.

You may also want to spray the solution on your carpets, sheets and washcloths, or pour one ounce in the washing machine as you do the laundry. Put it in your disposal to help disinfect the bacteria and mold and control odors.

Structured silver can be sprayed directly on vegetables or meats to help control E. coli and salmonella poisoning. It can also be used to disinfect jewelry or the baby's bed.

Human Papilloma Virus (HPV)

This is a viral infection usually afflicting the cervix. It destroys the cellular structure of the cells and can damage the DNA, causing cancer of the cervix.

> I used structured silver on Human Papillomavirus (HPV) warts. The patient had an outbreak around the rectum. He placed gel on warts for ten days. There was a 90 percent reduction of the HPV warts in ten days." – A certified Urologist

Most of the time there are no symptoms of HPV infection. The only way to know if you have HPV is to have lab tests performed by a doctor. No real treatment is given until the tissues damaged by the virus have become cancerous. At this point surgery is performed. If a woman uses a structured silver liquid (douche) and gel on a tampon she can destroy the virus that causes the abnormal cells, possibly preventing the cause of the cancer.

· Swallow two teaspoons of structured silver liquid twice a day for prevention and treatment.

· Apply structured silver gel to a tampon and insert into vagina for 90 minutes a day so the gel can stay in contact with germs in the vagina.

· To create a structured silver douche, use three ounces of structured silver liquid mixed with three ounces of distilled water. Pump the solution into the vaginal cavity and hold for ten minutes, then release. This should be done once a day, for five days, or until symptoms are gone.

· Take at least 8 billion active culture probiotic daily. Reduce dietary sugar and carbohydrates. And take large quantities of antioxidants daily. This will help neutralize and clear free radicals produced by pathogens.

Structured silver can destroy the virus that causes HPV in less than six minutes. Most women feel noticeably better in one day and may return to normal in as little as two to five days.

Hypertension (See High Blood Pressure)

Hypoglycemia

Hypoglycemia means low blood sugar. Hypoglycemic individuals experience spikes and drops in blood sugar, especially when eating something sugary. This fluctuation makes a person very susceptible to bacterial disease and makes healing difficult. Taking two teaspoons of structured silver twice a day and applying gel directly to wounds can experience improvements.

Immune Modulator

In HIV patients structured silver liquid was used 1 oz twice a day for four months and improved immune function an average of 40%. This means in an autoimmune and virus induced compromise, the structured silver liquid can improve the cellular number and reduced symptoms of the AIDS patients. In normal people the improvement is less but the over protection is greater.

Impetigo

Impetigo is a bacterial infection of the skin that shows up as blisters usually around the mouth. For prevention, drink one teaspoon of structured silver twice a day. If you already are suffering from impetigo, drink two teaspoons twice a day and, more importantly, apply the gel topically one to four times a day. When impetigo is kept moist with silver gel, it can spread less and improve much quicker. Since impetigo is contagious you will want to apply the structured silver gel to your hands as well in order to prevent contaminating yourself or others.

The first round of bottles has been used in about 85 patients consisting of adults and children, with great success for skin ulcers, fungus on the skin and nails, throat infections, tonsillitis, chicken pox and other skin bumps, badly infected cuts and wounds, ear infections, asthma and respiratory infections, and herpes. Everyone is very pleased, especially with the lack of side effects that strong antibiotics would have had. So the question is how can we get some more structured silver quickly!"
– From a letter from a ministry in Nicaragua that uses structured silver

Immune Support

Structured silver helps modulate immune response but its real benefit is that there are fewer germs afflicting the immune system. Since our germ-filled environment can overwork the immune system, it must prioritize its efforts. This means the immune system fights germs first, then builds and rebuilds tissue if it has the capacity to do so. By reducing the ever-present germ burden on an overworked immune system, the ability to heal increases significantly. People with autoimmune diseases can be confident in using structured silver on the skin and inside the body because it reduces inflammation, activates stem cells, and promotes normal healing.

Infant Health

Babies can use a lower dose of structured silver—half a normal adult dosage. The liquid and gel can be used on or in any orifice of the body. Infants 0-6 months old would take up to one-half teaspoon (of liquid silver) twice a day. Babies 6 months and older and weighing up to 75 pounds would take a dose of up to one teaspoon twice a day. Children over 75 pounds would take a normal adult dose of two teaspoons twice a day.

Infections, Bacterial (See antibacterial)

Infections, Viral (See antiviral)

Infectious Disease

Any time you are exposed to an infectious disease, you are at risk of having significant cellular, systemic, or tissue damage. It can also be fatal. To prevent the spread of infectious disease, apply silver gel to your hands every four hours. This will keep pathogens from getting on your face or in your eyes, and will prevent the transfer of disease to others. I recommend using a gel with a moisturizing agent like aloe so your skin doesn't dry out.

Inflammation and Swelling

Bacteria, viruses, parasites, or mold almost always cause inflammation. Structured silver can fight these causes. Drink two teaspoons twice daily and apply the gel to inflamed areas as needed. Sometimes an inflammatory response is found around an open wound like an MRSA or staph infection. In this case, spray the gel on the affected area twice daily.

Influenza (See Flu)

Inhaled Silver

Structured silver can be inhaled from a nebulizer (a nebulizer can be obtained at a medical supply store). The nebulizer creates a mist that you can inhale through a tube. This approach is very effective against bacteria, virus, and mold problems in the lungs and respiratory tract. Structured silver should be inhaled 30 minutes a day—15 minutes in the morning and evening, or 30 minutes at once. The liquid mist can destroy infections such as tuberculosis and pneumonia.

Intestinal Detox

Structured silver can help with intestinal detoxification. It can destroy yeast, bacterial, or viral infections. One hour after using a slippery elm product, cascara sagrada, laxative, or any other intestinal cleanse, use silver to remedy any infections.

Intravenous Treatment (IV) (See Cancer)

Irritable Bowel Syndrome (See Colitis)

Itching and Scaling

Itching and scaling can occur for many reasons, including bacteria, viruses, yeast, and allergies. Regardless of the cause, dry skin is always a factor. Structured silver gel or liquid will reduce pain, inflammation, itching, and scaling. Additionally, it may remove the cause of itching.

I went on a trip to Africa. I saw public advertisements all over the streets about treating fungal infections in the groin area. In Africa's warm, moist, tropical climate, this affects both men and women. People are making such extended use of gels, ointments, and antibiotics that their immune systems are being damaged. Individuals who applied structured silver gel found relief from itching in five minutes, with the redness and inflammation leaving in two hours.

Itching of the crotch is a common and embarrassing source of discomfort. This includes itchy vagina, itchy foreskin, itchy scrotum, and itchy rectum. For all of these itches, application of the gel several times a day can sooth the itch while simultaneously eliminating bacteria and fungus that may be the cause of the itch. Proper hygiene is essential for long-term prevention.

If you live in a warm, humid, or tropical climate, you may have a fungal or bacterial infection that grows in the warm, moist folds of the skin, including the groin. Simple application of the structured silver gel or liquid twice daily should keep it under control. For more aggressive cases, it can be used five times a day. In addition, at least one teaspoon of structured silver liquid should also be taken orally twice a day.

Structured silver can also be applied to itching behind the ears, itchy pimples, itchy armpits, and other areas affected by itch. The gel or liquid can be applied to children and adults of any age.

Joints (See Arthritis)

Keratosis

Many people have precancerous legions from sun damage on their shoulders, chest, and face. It presents itself as dry, flaky skin spots or small, reddened, inflamed areas on the skin for years before it becomes a skin cancer.

Structured silver gel can be applied topically once or twice a day, and one teaspoon of liquid silver can also be taken twice a day. I have seen a case of keratosis remedied in as little as two weeks. Treatment should generally be followed for at least two months.

Kidney Disease

Structured silver passes through the body totally unchanged and does not produce harmful metabolites. It will pass through the intestines, bloodstream, kidneys and urine, producing antibacterial and antiviral effects.

To help kidney disease, drink two teaspoons four times a day. (A smaller person will use one teaspoon four times a day.) This high dosage is necessary because it needs to pass through the kidney on a regular basis. As it passes through, it will disinfect and help bring the kidney infection under control in as little as 12 hours.

Lacerations

Taking two teaspoons twice daily of structured silver combined with a gel application four times daily can result in rapid recoveries without infection. The following is a quote from the Journal of Healing Outcomes on a patient who used a gel and liquid structured silver on a serious laceration. The following is a conclusion of why the structured silver works so successfully:

The topical application of structured silver gel kills pathogens and helps protect the wound from becoming contaminated or infected which means that the inflammatory phase of wound healing received significant assistance possibly by reducing the need for macrophages, monocytes and fewer cytokines producing less inflammatory response hormones. The fact that there is less inflammation suggests that there is a significant reduction in the inflammatory phase of healing.

Since the structured silver destroys bacteria, viruses and mold the wound was not infected, thus reducing the need for phagocytosis, which reduces the immune cascade required for clotting and decontamination of the wound. The elimination of bacteria leaves the wound edges and margins clean and capable of optimal healing. In addition there is an increased ability to secrete stem cells, which will produce multi-potent cellular healing. This produces obstacle-free wound healing, making a cleaner-healing scar. This can be seen in the fact that the wound was closed and stitches removed by day three where the wound presented a very low amount of inflammation, with no bacterial contamination. This could help explain why there is very little scarring. This could also be due to the fact that with less inflammation, there is less need for the platelets to produce histamine, cytokines and prostaglandins, which results in less overall swelling. This means the wound can heal faster because there are less factors competing with collagen. This reduced inflammation results in more collagen filling the fibrin - fibronectin matrix producing less tension, better bridging to migrate across the wound and less constriction (fibrotic scarring of the wound).

In addition the gel provides a wound that is moist promoting the migration of polymorphonuclear cells stretching across the wound, which can lay the foundation of a healthy uncomplicated wound. In addition it appears that stem cell activation (as published in Nexus 2008), could be responsible for the rapid adhesion of the laceration and assist in the removal of the scab and reduction of the scarring. This could occur because the endothelialization had less opposition from bacteria, mold and inflammation.

It appears that stem cells had activated and mobilized angiogenesis from the healthy blood vessels as evidenced by the pink coloration of the tissues immediately surrounding the suture lines, which indicate that stem-cell-activated angiogenesis had taken place with remarkable results, probably due to the fact that there was no bacterial infection nor any contamination and its associative inflammation.

In short, the structured silver appears to play a significant role to decontaminate, prevent infection and stimulate stem cells, resulting in improved wound healing characterized by reduced inflammation, improved angiogenesis, more efficient phagocytosis and reduced scarring.

Since there is less need for polymorphonulclear cells there will be fewer helper

T cells secreting cytokines that cause the multiplication of inflammatory factors. This means there is less cleanup of inflammation and the wound in general. In addition there will be better stem cell production from the healthy fringes of the blood vessels, better collagen production and improved circulation due to the fact that vasodilation and blood vessel permeability will be normalized sooner in an uninfected and less inflamed wound. All of these parameters seem to have one thing in common: structured silver has antimicrobial abilities that help reduce infection, and inflammation resulting in better healing. Since inflammation lasts as long as there is debris or infection in the wound, it can be said that structured silver can help remove the cause of a significant amount of infection and inflammation. This results in improved healing outcomes by reducing the pathogenic burden on the immune system, allowing optimal restorative and regenerative immune functions.

Leukemia

Leukemia is a cancer of the blood or bone marrow and is characterized by an abnormal proliferation of blood cells, usually white blood cells. Structured silver can help with leukemia by drinking four ounces for two days, sipping it every hour. Drink two ounces a day for the next five days. Drink two tablespoons in the morning and at night for maintenance. Remember milk thistle to help cleanse the liver, antioxidants to help cleanse the bloodstream.

Leprosy

Leprosy is bacteria that have become resistant to antibiotics. In Biblical times, it was the worst contagious disease in existence. Those suffering from it were quarantined to leper colonies. It may surprise you to know that there are still leper colonies today in Hawaii, India and other places around the world.

Structured silver can destroy leprosy. By drinking two teaspoons two to three times a day and applying structured silver gel topically three times a day, you can fight even the most serious leprosy wounds. Lepers have been able to bring their disease under control within two days using structured silver.

Leichmaniasis

Leichmaniasis is a parasitic infection. It shows up just under the skin as a purple rash and raises welts and boil-like symptoms all over the body. Soldiers in Afghanistan have been suffering from this infection and it has been very difficult to remedy.

The army hospital at William Beaumont Army Medical Hospital conducted a study on leichmaniasis, using structured silver liquid and gel. They found that drinking two teaspoons two to three times a day could destroy the parasite. The gel should also be applied two to four times as needed. You can expect to see a benefit over the course of eight weeks.

Lips

Many people suffer from chapped lips, the herpes virus (cold sores), or the lead in their lipstick. Placing silver gel on the lips every night will help to improve the lips and help to prevent damage. In addition, drink one teaspoon of structured silver liquid twice a day.

Lip Balm

It is easy to create your own silver lip balm. By adding a little bit of heat, you can melt your preferred lip balm. Add a small amount of liquid silver and then let the balm re-thicken. This will allow you to enjoy the benefits of silver each time you moisten your lips.

Liver Disease (see also Hepatitis)

The liver is one of the most important organs of the body. It detoxifies the blood and secretes over 4,000 enzymes. When the liver is inflamed, as in the case of hepatitis, it won't secrete as many enzymes and the blood will not be purified as quickly.

Structured silver can destroy the bacteria and viruses that harm the liver. By restoring proper liver function, all systems of the body are benefited, and overall wellness is increased. For these results, drink two tablespoons of structured silver twice daily. For severe cases of hepatitis, this amount should be doubled.

Lung Disease

Cigarette smoke, toxins, and bacterial or viral infections can damage our lungs. Structured silver has been shown to destroy tuberculosis in laboratory testing. The lungs can be helped from both the inside and outside by drinking two teaspoons of structured silver daily and inhaling from a nebulizer 15 minutes twice a day.

Structured silver can also be put in a humidifier and used while sleeping at night. For serious conditions, structured silver may also be taken intravenously.

Lupus

Lupus is an autoimmune disease that can affect various parts of the body, including the skin, joints, heart, lungs, blood, kidneys, and brain. Because it is an autoimmune disease, you can't use major immune stimulation products. Structured silver can be used to the kill bacteria, viruses, mold, and parasites that may be the cause of the lupus. It will do this without making the lupus symptoms worse.

Structured silver can be of benefit when you drink one teaspoon three times a day. It can also be applied topically to facial rashes commonly caused by lupus. In addition, you can use acidophilus, antioxidants, coenzyme Q10, and an intestinal cleanse.

Lyme Disease

Lyme disease is caused by the bacteria Borrelia burgdorferi. It is primarily transmitted to humans by the bite of infected ticks belonging to a few species of the genus Ixodes ("hard ticks"). Lyme disease can also come from infected mice, horses, dogs, cattle, birds and rodents. It is the most common vector-borne disease in the United States.

Clinical manifestations of Lyme disease are divided into three stages: 1. Flu-like symptoms and a bulls-eye type of skin rash (erythema migrans). 2. Weeks or months later, Bells palsy or meningitis-type of neurologic symptoms develop. 3. Months to years later, arthritis develops. Symptoms get progressively worse if the cause of the disease is not eliminated.

Physicians usually prescribe antibiotics such as doxycycline, ceftriax-one, or amoxicillin. These seem to be fairly effective against Lyme disease if given within the first two weeks of infection, but the efficacy may diminish over time due to the progressive nature of the disease.

Ticks feed once during each of their three stages of life: larval ticks feed in late summer, nymphs in the following spring, and adults during the fall. Most human infections occur during the summer months. Under laboratory conditions the tick was required to feed for 24-36 hours or longer to transmit infections. This means that a human must have the infected tick feeding on them for two days in order to get infected. So the first line of defense against Lyme disease is to spread structured silver gel on high-risk areas of the skin on a daily basis. This daily surveillance should prevent the tick from infecting the skin for a 36-hour period.

If you think you have been bitten by a tick within the past two weeks, drink two ounces of liquid structured silver a day and apply gel to the bite four times a day for two weeks.

If you have Lyme disease, drink two ounces of structured silver liquid twice a day and apply gel to affected or sore areas twice a day. Continue this for three months, then reduce the dose by half for a month and return to full dose for a month and continue as long as needed. The reason to alternate high and low doses is because the bacterium drills down into muscle and hides from treatment, but rises up out of the muscle when not attacked so a high dose can be more effective a month later.

Note: Some people who have a difficult case of Lyme disease may want to drink eight ounces of structured silver at one time to initiate this treatment.

For prevention of Lyme disease, drink two teaspoons of structured silver liquid twice a day and apply structured silver gel twice a day.

Lymphatics

Lymphatics are used to cleanse the lymph system. The lymph system is parallel to the circulatory system in that it has glands in all the major circulatory areas. But the lymph system does not have a heart or a pump attached to it. The movement of the body controls lymph flow.

Since the lymph is only circulated when the body moves, it is essential to walk, move your arms, stretch, and exercise to make your lymph system circulate out all of the toxins. A sore throat, for example, occurs when the lymph glands gather bacteria that are being circulated through the lymph, into the circulatory system, and out of the body.

I traveled to Ghana, where we gave liquid structured silver to children with malaria. We saw even the most severe cases remedied in five days. These children continued to follow the treatment for 10 days.

I saw one two-year-old child who was literally hours away from death, suffering from ear and throat infections and fever associated with malaria. Within four days of using silver he was completely healthy.

To help the lymph system do its job of getting the toxins and bacteria out of the body, drink two teaspoons of structured silver twice a day and apply the gel to affected areas twice a day.

Malaria

Swallow two ounces of liquid structured silver every day for two weeks and apply structured silver gel four times a day to wounds (if necessary). For prevention swallow two teaspoons twice a day and apply gel as needed.

Makeup Base

Structured silver can be used in addition to, or in place of, makeup base. After you wash your face, apply a thin layer of structured silver gel. Wait two minutes for it to dry and then apply your base. This will give you protection against acne, blemishes, and infections from mold, bacteria, and viruses.

Some women use the structured silver gel as their base and natural coloring. This approach can replace damaging makeup and allergenic topic cleansing, as it washes clean with water.

Makeup Irritation

When people put on makeup everyday it often begins to irritate their skin. The skin may become red and itchy and rashes can form. To neutralize this problem, apply structured silver gel and drink structured silver liquid on a daily basis.

One teaspoon of silver liquid should be taken twice daily. In addition, when the makeup is removed, soak a cotton ball with silver and wipe the face clean. This will neutralize pathogens that may aggravate or irritate the skin. It will also help with pain, redness, and skin regeneration.

To add another layer of protection, structured silver should also be applied at night before bed. Hypoallergenic makeup will also prevent irritation problems.

Massage Therapists and Other Health Care Professionals (for Protection)

Massage therapists have one great enemy, infection. The patients bring infections on their skin in the form of acne, rashes, staph, blisters, streptococcus, and yeast. These are highly contagious and can be spread from patient to therapist. Some of the infectious agents like MRSA (methicillin-resistant Staphylococcus aureus) can be transferred by touch and can infect the patient, therapist and surrounding environment, leaving everyone who enters the room at risk of a potentially fatal infection. There are hundreds of therapists that have contacted MRSA from their patients. I recommend structured silver for massage therapists and all other medical professionals who come in contact with skin. They should use it for self-protection as well as protection for their patients.

- Apply structured silver gel to any at-risk regions of the skin, nose, eyes, face or other exposed skin areas as often as needed (usually 1-10 times a day).
- Drink two teaspoons of structured silver liquid twice a day.

Memory Enhancement

Memory can be negatively impacted by bacteria-caused inflammation. Structured silver can help reduce the inflammation by drinking two teaspoons twice a day. By inhaling silver from a nebulizer, it can go straight to the brain. Inhale 15 minutes a day for memory enhancement and 30 minutes for infectious issues.

Phosphatidylserine, coenzyme Q10, ginkgo biloba, and B-complex vitamins can help as well.

Menopause

Menopause is the complete shutting down of the female reproductive system. Structured silver make hot flashes less significant by fighting bacterial, viral, or vaginal yeast infections. It also reduces the aches and pains associated with menopause. The liquid can be taken every day, one teaspoon twice a day, or as needed. The gel can be applied to any painful area of the body, including the breasts.

Migraine Headaches (See Headaches)

Mold and Fungus

Fungus and mold grow in warm, moist, and sugared areas such as the intestines or vagina. Taking sugar out of your diet and using silver both topically and internally can treat these. Take two teaspoons of silver three times a day and apply it topically one to four times a day, if needed. This dosage should be continued for at least two weeks longer than symptoms are present.

You can expect to see a benefit within the first 30 minutes. It will take at least 10 minutes for the liquid to kill a fungal infection on the skin. Silver will work best when taken with complementary products such as probiotics, caprylic acid, anti-yeast diets, essential fatty acids, and amino acids.

Silver can also be sprayed on household items. In about 10 minutes it will kill the fungus, bacteria, or viruses on your table, food, clothes, phone, refrigerator, or toilet.

Mononucleosis

Mononucleosis is an infection that produces flu-like symptoms. To relieve the symptoms, drink four ounces for two days, sipping every hour. Drink two ounces a day for the next five days. For maintenance, drink two tablespoons in the morning and at night. Use topically as needed.

Mouth Wash

Dental floss can be used in combination with the mouthwash. It will prevent infection if you pour 2 tablespoons of the liquid structured silver into the dental floss container and floss with silver soaked string.

Morgellons

Morgellons is a disease that presents itself in many ways, but all of them involve inflammation, swelling tissue damage and dry, flaky, pustulant skin rashes. Some believe it is caused by a parasite, and others think it is caused by a fungus. In either case the solution can be structured silver, which destroys bacteria, viruses and yeast.

Apply the gel as often as needed to keep the skin moist because it seems to heal better when it is not dry and flaky. Drink two tablespoons of the liquid twice a day. In cases where the skin is extremely dry and flaky, a moisturizing product like aloe vera mixed with the structured silver to keep skin moist can be used.

Note: A moist wound is important to minimize the rash but a wound that is too wet will become macerated.

MRSA and Staph

MRSA (Methycillin-resistant Staphylococcus aureus) is a resistant variation of the common bacterium Staphylococcus aureus. The organism is resistant to a significant group of antibiotics called the beta lactase, which includes penicillins. MRSA is approaching pandemic levels. There is an immediate need for a substance like structured silver in controlling this potentially fatal disease. According to the Journal of the American Medical Association (58), MRSA was responsible for 94,360 serious infections and associated with 18,650 hospital-stay-related deaths in the United States in 2005. The statistics suggest that MRSA infections are responsible for more deaths in the U.S. each year than AIDS.

Symptoms of MRSA usually manifest as a patch of small pustules surrounded by redness and swelling. It may resemble a pimple, spider bite, or boil and may not be accompanied by a fever. The bumps become larger and spread and these larger pus-filled boils can develop deep into the tissue. Most cases infect the skin; a minority of these infections can invade vital organs and cause sepsis, toxic shock syndrome, flesh eating (necrotizing) and pneumonia.

· Drink two tablespoons of structured silver liquid three times a day. This is triple times the normal dose and will work nicely if taken as needed until symptoms subside.

- Apply silver gel to the affected area and surrounding tissue 2-6 times a day. Currently structured silver is the only prophylactic that has activity against MRSA. It can be used for prevention as well as treatment of MRSA. It is important to note that daily use of structured silver does not produce resistant strains of MRSA.

> My son was on the wrestling team in high school. He got an MRSA infection from the wrestling mat, they say. He missed school for a month and could not wrestle because he had a contagious rash. It was eating his flesh. The antibiotics helped but could not get rid of it. He started using silver—drinking two tablespoons twice a day and putting the gel on his rash twice a day. He got better in three weeks and is now wrestling again. The coach now sprays the mat with structured silver every day and gave a tube of gel to every team member. I find that families are using it at home too.

Multiple Sclerosis

Multiple sclerosis (MS) is an autoimmune condition in which the immune system attacks the central nervous system. Structured silver can impact it dramatically when you drink two tablespoons, three times a day and inhale structured silver 15 minutes a day.

By drinking liquid structured silver, the silver gets into circulation and can get to the base of the brain stem. By inhaling, it will reach the brain stem a bit quicker. This will prevent the secondary effects associated with multiple sclerosis. In addition, arginine, coenzyme Q10, B-complex vitamins, and lesafin can benefit MS.

Myocardial Infarction

Myocardial infarction (MI) is a condition where the heart often stops beating and is usually caused by the clogging of heart arteries. This usually begins with problems in the mouth and gums.

To kill the bacteria in the mouth, one ounce of liquid structured silver should be held in the mouth for six minutes and then swallowed. By doing this daily, you can destroy the bacteria that causes damage to the heart and heart valves.

Neck Firming Cream

When a person ages, the skin can stretch due to the loss of elastin and collagen.

By applying structured silver topically to the neck, you can remove the fungus and bacteria that may reside in the dead skin cells or wrinkles of the neck. The wrinkles will stop growing deeper and you will have a more youthful-looking skin. In this way you'll have better skin texture. To achieve these benefits, put silver gel in the refrigerator, take it out, and apply while cold 1-4 times a day.

Nerves

Nerves transmit electrical and chemical energy, directing the movement of the body. Any inflammatory disease will inflame the tissues, which can put pressure on the nerves and send pain throughout the body. Structured silver can reduce inflammation, pain, and pressure on the nerves.

Two teaspoons of liquid silver can be taken internally daily. Structured silver gel can also be applied to the affected areas to help reduce inflammation and pain associated with nerves problems.

Night Cream

You might want to mix your toner or moisturizing cream with structured silver to produce an antibacterial toner or moisturizer. The moisturizer would require you to pour out 20% of the moisturizer and replace it with structured silver liquid. Shake well and use to prevent pathogens while moisturizing. The same percentages work for toners (20% structured silver liquid with 80% toner).

Nose and Sinuses

Nose and sinus congestion can stop you from breathing properly. Congestion leads to high production of mucus and can clog the nose, throat, sinuses, and lungs. If bacteria cause the congestion, it can last for months if is not destroyed.

By applying three or four sprays of liquid structured silver intranasally, you will protect the nose and sinuses from developing a bacterial, viral, or fungal infection. This should be done two to four times a day. In addition, drink one teaspoon of structured silver twice a day. This will reduce sinusitis, colds, and other problems associated with nasal congestion.

Nose Drops

Using an intranasal sprayer (nasal atomizer) or dropper, you can pump structured silver liquid into your sinuses. You can also tip your head back and use silver as nose drops. This allows the liquid to flow through your sinuses. You will feel it flow out on the back or your throat, where it will help detoxify the sinuses and throat.

Many people get recurring sore throats from postnasal drip, which is when mucus drips from the sinuses into the back of the throat. Nasal drops and nasal spray will help remedy postnasal drip and congestion.

Obesity

Structured silver does not burn fat, thus it does not change obesity. Obesity compresses arteries, nerves, the stomach, and the overall amount of fats in the intestines. This causes circulatory, hormonal, and intestinal problems.

Drinking two teaspoons of structured silver twice a day and using it topically as needed can help with some of the problems associated with obesity. The silver can destroy excess yeast in the intestines. It can also reduce scarring caused by stretch marks. Digestive and liver cleansing and milk thistle should be used in combination with the structured silver when targeting obesity.

Orifices

Structured silver can be used in any orifice of the body—eyes, ears, nose, mouth, rectum, or vagina.

Osteoporosis

Osteoporosis is a disease of bone that leads to an increased risk of fracture. Though structured silver will not help with the thinning of the bone, it will help with wound healing by reducing the fungus, bacteria, and mold that may otherwise inhibit healing. Using calcium, magnesium, and vitamin D twice a day will also help.

Pain

Pain is a very important tool for diagnosing disease. Most people don't even think about checking themselves for an illness or getting treatment until they feel pain.

Silver gel can be used topically to reduce mild and moderate pain. Drinking one teaspoon of liquid silver each day may also help. If the pain persists, you should visit the doctor to see if there is a problem. Using antioxidants and stretching will also reduce pain.

Pancreas

Pancreas problems cause blood sugar to get out of balance, leading to diabetes and depression. Pancreatitis is caused by a viral or bacterial infection, usually from bad food or water. Because pancreas issues can escalate quickly, it is important to take structured silver on a regular basis, drinking two teaspoons twice a day.

Parasites

The World Health Organization estimates that one in four people have a chronic parasitic infection of some kind. It may be in the intestines, under the skin, or in the lungs. Parasites can come from the food we eat, including pork and fish. Once they are inside our bodies, they lay eggs. The eggs hatch and take up residence in the body, and then the process is repeated. It is important to get rid of parasites permanently.

Structured silver can help. It does not kill all parasites, but it does help in the intestines, in the blood, and with leichmaniasis. Structured silver will need to be used for three months, as the lifecycle of each generation of parasites is about 45 days. During this time, drink two teaspoons twice a day. Black walnut hulls, digestive cleansing, and milk thistle will also help this process.

Parkinson's Disease

Parkinson's Disease is a degenerative disorder of the central nervous system that often impairs the sufferer's motor skills and speech, as well as other functions. Brain inflammation is also associated with the disease. By drinking structured silver two teaspoons twice daily and taking methylsulfanyl methane (MSM) twice daily, the toxicity and inflammation inside of the brain may be reduced. B-complex vitamins, lecatin, and phosphatidyl seri will also help. With this treatment you should see improvement beginning in the first two weeks and continuing over the next two months.

Pelvic Inflammatory Disease

Pelvic inflammatory disease refers to chronic inflammation of the pelvic region due to ongoing infections. Symptoms of pelvic inflammatory disease usually include long-term inflammation and infections of the vagina, vulva, uterus, and surrounding tissues. Pain may be present for a short or long period of time and is aggravated by urination, sexual activity or yeast overgrowth. Nausea and fever may also be present.

Bacteria, viruses, and yeast infections usually cause pelvic inflammatory disease.

- Swallow two teaspoons of structured silver liquid twice a day for prevention. Drink two tablespoons twice a day for severe conditions.
- Apply silver gel topically to affected and painful area at least twice a day to destroy the pathogens that cause the pain and infection.
- To create a structured silver douche, mix three ounces of liquid silver liquid with

three ounces of distilled water. Pump the solution into the vaginal cavity and hold for ten minutes, then release. This should be done once a day, for five days, or until symptoms are gone.

· As an optional use, pour four ounces of silver liquid into a full tub of warm water. Soak and relax, flushing the silver water into the vaginal cavity. Twenty-five minutes is average for a muscle relaxing vaginal flush in the tub.

Personal Lubricant

Personal lubricant can be used to lubricate joints of the elbow or armpit, or anywhere skin is rubbing together and causing a rash.

It is most commonly used, however, on condoms or for vaginal dryness. By using silver gel as a personal lubricant, you will destroy bacteria, viruses, and mold—protecting both yourself and your sexual partner. It will also reduce the inflammation, swelling, and pain associated with skin rubbing against skin.

Pet Use

You can use structured silver liquid or gel for your pet. If a pet weighs 20 pounds, it should receive one fourth of the human dosage. In most cases, pets take one fourth to one sixth of the normal human dose, but they can safely take up to quadruple doses when they have a problem.

Pneumonia

Pneumonia is an inflammatory illness of the lung and is caused by both viruses and bacteria. The lungs can become so filled with fluid that asphyxiation occurs. Structured silver can destroy the bacteria or the viral infection that causes pneumonia. The recommended dosage is two teaspoons, two to four times a day; 15 minutes of inhalation from a nebulizer; and intranasal spray twice a day to reduce congestion. You should expect to see benefits in the first 12 hours. In severe cases an IV protocol is an option (see also Cancer)

Post-Surgical

Surgery opens the possibility of infection in wounds, stitches, and incisions. Hospital-acquired methicillin-resistant staph aureus infections (MRSA) are one of the most dangerous infections you can get. Structured silver gel should be applied to the wound, stitches, and the surrounding area immediately after surgery. This will prevent infection, help wound healing, and reduce scarring.

Poultice

Silver gel can be placed on a body part and then wrapped in place as a poultice. This allows the wound to remain uncontaminated and to improve quicker. Silver poultice has been used in horses for years to treat infections. It can be mixed with any other desired herbs.

Prostate Disease

The prostate is the gland that closes off the flow of urine from the bladder. When the prostate relaxes, urine will flow out of the bladder and into the toilet. The prostate gland then tightens back up on the ureter and stops the urine flow. Over time, the prostate muscle becomes bigger. If it becomes infected with bacteria, it will swell and become too large and shut off the flow of urine, making you unable to urinate.

Structured silver can destroy the bacteria that cause the prostatitis. By drinking two teaspoons twice a day you will have enough circulating in your system to go through your urine and kill the bacteria in your bladder and prostate. Some people have felt a benefit by placing the gel between the rectum and scrotum. Using saw palmetto twice a day should also reduce inflammation in the prostate. For those who have access to a catheter, 2 oz of liquid silver can be pumped directly into the catheter and into the bladder for ten minutes where it will kill pathogens.

Psoriasis

Psoriasis is a disorder that affects the skin and joints. It commonly causes red scaly patches to appear on the skin. This condition makes you very susceptible to secondary bacterial infection getting into the cracked areas of the skin.

To fight the bacteria, apply structured silver gel two to four times a day, keeping skin, wounds, or rashes very moist. Drink one teaspoon of structured silver liquid twice daily. For very dry, scaly skin, silver liquid and gel can be mixed with Vaseline (one part gel, liquid, and Vaseline). This will keep the affected areas moisturized for a much longer period of time. Using a structured silver gel with aloe will help with the most difficult situations, including Morgellon's disease.

Pus

Pus is produced when bacteria break down and destroy healthy cells. Apply silver gel topically to affected areas one to four times a day and drink two teaspoons of structured silver twice a day. If pus is being produced in your throat, e.g. sore throat or strep throat, rinse your mouth with structured silver liquid or apply gel to the throat. Try to keep in place for 6 minutes.

Pyorrhea (Gum Disease)

In addition to causing bad breath, gum disease erodes the gums and bones around the teeth, causing the teeth to fall out. Rinsing your mouth with one ounce of structured silver six minutes each day can prevent gum disease—the remaining rinse should be swallowed. You may also brush your teeth with a silver gel. Coenzyme Q10 will also be of benefit.

You can expect to have a benefit after the first brushing of your teeth. After three days you will have noticeable improvement.

Rashes

Rashes can occur on any part of the body. They can come from irritation or chemicals that irritate. By putting silver gel with aloe right on the rash, you will moisturize, detoxify, and quicken healing. Apply one to four times a day and swallow one teaspoon of structured silver liquid twice a day.

Razor Burn

By shaving, you cut off microscopic pieces of skin, causing razor burn. Structured silver gel can be used as shaving cream or you can wash your face with structured silver liquid immediately after shaving.

Shaving with acne usually results in small open wounds. In this case, you should wet your face with water, and then shave using structured silver gel and a razor. When you're finished, rinse off the gel and apply a thin layer of either structured silver liquid or gel. The wounds will improve quicker and the bacteria will die off faster. You can expect to see a benefit after the first day.

Reproductive Organs, Male

Men who have not been circumcised tend to have more hygiene problems than those who have. Uncircumcised men can apply structured silver gel under the foreskin to help stop fungal, bacterial, and viral infections.

Respiratory Health

Respiratory health problems are a common ailment for many of us. A virus generally causes colds, the flu, bronchitis, and asthma. Structured silver can help destroy these viruses. To prevent exposure to germs on an airplane, spray silver into

A few years ago, AIDS was spreading very rapidly in some Southeast Asian countries. The World Health Organization did a study to find the cause. It discovered that the virus was being stored under the foreskin of uncircumcised men and then being passed to the partner during intercourse.

To prevent the spread of disease, circumcision was made mandatory. The rate of AIDS was reduced by 95 percent in one year. Legal rulings in these countries found these mandatory circumcisions to be unlawful, and the requirement was repealed. Within three years, the number of AIDS cases was as high as it had been previously.

Structured silver can significantly help uncircumcised men from transmitting disease.

your nose. Before you go to a nursery, swallow, rinse, or brush your teeth with silver gel. Use hand gel to prevent the transfer of contagious disease from hands to the face or eyes.

Germs are not the only cause of disease. An air conditioner or heater that is set too high, or on for too long, can dry out the air. This will dry out your nose, throat, and lungs. If they become chapped or cracked, viruses can enter very easily. Conversely, some homes or offices are too humid. Fungus or black mold grows in warm, moist areas including your lungs and sinuses. To avoid either of these problems, a preventative dose should be sprayed into the nose every day.

Rosacea

Rosacea is a form of bacteria that grows on the nose, making it red and swollen with pimples. This can leave very large scars. Because it is difficult to treat, doctors generally prescribe antibiotics.

Rather than use antibiotics, you can drink two teaspoons structured silver liquid twice a day and apply gel four times a day. Wash the nose lightly between each application. You should see a reduction of redness within the first two hours and a reduction of pimples in the first day.

Scalp Treatment

Men who shave their head can apply structured silver gel to the head to prevent razor burn. Placing a structured silver gel with aloe on your scalp every night after washing will keep it moisturized and prevent it from flaking or having sun damage spots. Repeating this process twice a day will also improve the texture of your skin.

Women can use the solution to remedy hair loss caused by bacteria. Structured silver can also help with dry scalp. Spray one to two ounces into wet hair and rub it in. Let stand for 10 minutes before rinsing.

Scars

A scar is formed when the skin is damaged and the immune system pulls it back together. The scar is made up of thickened layers of skin. Drinking one teaspoon of structured silver liquid twice a day and applying structured silver gel directly to the wound two to four times a day can minimize scarring. The silver will keep the wound moist and remove bacteria, mold, and viruses and help the improvement process.

Structured silver gel can also be applied directly to scars and stretch marks, softening the skin and reducing scar size. For severe, highly inflamed, or keloid scars, apply the gel and cover it with plastic wrap or a sterile gauze bandage.

Sinusitis (See Nose and Sinuses)

Sitz Bath

For people who don't have the ability to get in and out of a tub, structured silver can be used as a spray or poured on a washcloth as a Sitz bath. By washing with a washcloth and drying with a dry towel, you can detoxify warm, moist areas that may grow yeast.

Skin Cleanse

Cleansing the skin is very simple. Wash the skin with a mild, hypoallergenic mild soap, pat it dry and while the skin is still moist, apply structured silver gel. Drink one teaspoon of silver liquid twice a day for prevention.

If you have open wounds, you should apply gel more regularly. If the wound is a MRSA infection, apply silver gel every two hours to keep it moist.

According to the Surgeons Scrub Test protocol, structured silver gel was found to kill 99.999 percent of all pathogens, bacteria, virus, and mold for a total of four hours.

Structured silver can also be combined with other bar or pump soaps. By heating a bar of soap and adding liquid silver, you can create a soap that has the benefits of silver. Mixing silver with pump soap gives the same benefit.

Skin Conditioner

Structured silver makes a perfect skin conditioner because it does not contain alcohol or greasy petroleum products. To moisturize skin, apply the liquid or gel after you wash your face and before applying makeup.

Skin Damage

Skin can be damaged by many things, including wind, sun, makeup, and detergent. To keep it healthy, we need a protective barrier. The protective barrier usually comes from oils that are secreted from our skin. But as we get older we secrete less and less of these protective oils. By using structured silver on the skin one to four times a day, the skin will stay moist and a protective antibacterial barrier will be created to prevent disease from entering the skin.

My daughter is a performer who sings in front of thousands of people each night. When she travels to different cities she is exposed to cigarette smoke, pollution, and lack of sleep. These factors, combined with her singing, often result in a throat that is overworked.

To soothe her throat, we created a throat spray that consisted of a mixture of structured silver liquid, essential oils, and a little bit of glycerin. After spraying it in the back of her throat, she found immediate relief. The voice box was lubricated and the structured silver destroyed bacteria, viruses, and mold and reduced inflammation. She was then able to sing for longer periods of time without damaging her throat.

Skin Softening

For skin to soften, it must be moist and receive necessary nutrients. To soften skin, apply a structured silver gel with aloe vera topically one to four times a day and in ingest structured silver liquid one teaspoon twice a day.

Sore Throat

A sore throat is generally caused by bacteria, but may also be a result of a virus. To kill the bacteria that cause puss, swollen tonsils, and red spots in the back of your throat, rinse your mouth with one ounce of structured silver for six minutes. Allow a small amount of the solution to trickle down the back of your throat and swallow every 30 seconds. Swallow the remainder when you're done. Pump structured silver into your nasal cavity as needed for sore throat, congestion, or postnasal drip. Sinuses and throat need to be treated simultaneously so one does not infect the other.

Stomachache

If you have a stomachache and you don't know what is causing it, structured silver can usually help. By taking one ounce of silver liquid every hour for four hours, bacterial or viral infections can quickly be resolved.

Stress

Any single item, even imagined worries, can cause stress. Silver can reduce the stressful impact of bacteria, viruses, and mold on all the systems of the body. By reducing the stress, the immune system has less trouble to deal with and you will be sick less often.

Stretch Marks (See Scars)

Stroke

Stoke is a circulatory issue that takes place inside the brain. Silver liquid can help by destroying the bacteria or viruses that can cause inflammation in the circulatory system. When used after a stroke, structured silver can quicken the removal of blood pooled in the brain. These benefits can come by drinking two teaspoons of silver twice a day. It can also be inhaled in nebulized form.

Substance Abuse

Structured silver gel can be applied to injection sites, abscesses, skin rashes or traumatic injuries caused by substance abuse. Swallow two teaspoons twice a day of liquid silver and apply structured silver gel 2-10 times a day to injured areas.

Sunburn (See burns)

Suppository Use

The use of special structured silver suppositories can be very effective at delivering silver into the bloodstream. By placing a suppository into the rectum, the colon can absorb hundreds of times more structured silver nanoparticles into the bloodstream. This phenomenon occurs because structured silver doesn't have to pass through acid in the stomach. Stomach acid binds with silver and serves to slow absorption. The rectal delivery of structured silver can be achieved by using a special structured silver suppository or by pushing one teaspoon of structured silver gel into the rectum twice a day.

Thyroid

The thyroid gland is the major gland for the hormone system of the body. Damage to this gland can result in lack of energy, too much energy, weight gain, or weight loss. Structured silver can help because often the thyroid is damaged by a viral or bacterial infection. Drinking two teaspoons twice a day and applying structured silver gel to the throat will result in significant thyroid benefit.

Toenail Fungus

When structured silver comes in contact with toenail fungus, it can kill it within minutes. The problem is getting underneath the nail. If possible, get through the nail and clear out as much fungus as possible with a blunt instrument. Soaking the toe in structured silver for 30 minutes every other day can then treat the toenail fungus.

If you can't get the structured silver through the nail, file down the top layer of the nail until it becomes water-soluble. This will allow the silver to reach the fungus and kill it. It will take several months for the nail to grow out completely.

Tonic

Structured silver can be used as a tonic. It helps the liver to improve itself, function better, and produce more healthy enzymes by cleaning out the bacteria, viruses, and mold. This will also result in more energy. Drink two teaspoons one to four times a day, or as needed.

Tonsillitis

Tonsillitis is the inflammation of the tonsils. It's almost always caused by bacteria. Once it begins, it often has to be resolved surgically. This is unfortunate because tonsils are a key organ in the immune system.

By rinsing with one ounce of liquid silver for six minutes each day, you will kill the bacteria. This process can be repeated daily for a very serious tonsillitis flare up. Spraying silver into the nostrils will also help. The more contact the silver has with the back of the throat, the faster it will work.

Toothache (See cavities)

Toothpaste

Using silver gel as toothpaste will allow you to brush away bacteria, viruses, and mold as well as destroy bad breath. It can be mixed half and half with your regular toothpaste, if desired.

Tongue

The tongue can suffer from a number of maladies, including canker sores and bacterial and viral infections. Whatever the cause of the problem, you should rinse with one ounce of liquid structured silver for six minutes twice a day.

If you have a white pasty substance on your tongue, it's likely a yeast infection. You may want to brush your tongue with structured silver gel in addition to the rinse. For cankers, you can also apply structured silver gel directly to the tongue.

Tuberculosis

Tuberculosis is a common and often deadly infectious disease caused by mycobacteria. Structured silver has destroyed tuberculosis in laboratory studies. By drinking two teaspoons twice daily and inhaling from a nebulizer 30 minutes each day, you may affect the tuberculosis in both the lungs and the bloodstream.

Tuberculosis is not easy to beat. This dosage of structured silver may need to be followed for weeks or months. You should see benefits after the first dose and each repeated use.

Ulcers

Ulcers are caused by a bacterium called H. pylori. It destroys the lining of the stomach and intestines, sometimes causing a bleeding ulcer. By drinking one teaspoon of silver three to five times a day, it can enter the stomach and destroy the bacteria causing the ulcer.

It should take two weeks to get the H. pylori under control, but treatment should be continued for at least a month. H. pylori can return just by having poor hygiene, eating out at restaurants, or not washing your hands. Using silver gel can prevent its spread.

Urinary Tract Infection (UTI)

A urinary infection (UTI) is bacterial infection that affects any part of the urinary tract. The kidney, ureters and bladder are adversely affected by an invading bacterium and multiply in the urine.

The most common symptoms of a UTI are pain and burning during urination, more frequent urination, and an abnormal urgency to urinate without vaginal discharge.

Bacteria, viruses and fungus that infect the genital area cause UTI's.

· Drink two ounces of silver liquid every hour for four hours. Since structured silver destroys the bacteria that cause the infection in six minutes, it is important to absorb large amounts of silver for four hours. In this way the structured silver can wash through the kidneys and pool in the bladder. Structured silver passes through the body unchanged so the part that pools in the bladder will still kill bacteria in the kidneys, bladder and urethra.

· Apply structured silver gel topically twice a day to affected area, or as needed.
· Take at least 8 billion active probiotic cultures that contain acidophilus and bifidus daily.
· Take large doses of antioxidants. This will help neutralize and clear free radicals produced by pathogens.
· Cranberry is terrific at helping reduce bladder infections.

Structured silver can destroy bacteria that cause infections in the urinary tract in under six minutes. This means you can expect the liquid and gel to destroy the cause of the UTI as long as the structured silver stays in contact with the pathogen for six minutes. Most women feel noticeably better in two hours and may return to normal in as little as four to six hours.

> I have been troubled by yeast infections and bacterial infections for twenty years. Recently I have been using structured silver gel twice a day on my female areas when I have sex, as a personal lubricant. I have not had a single yeast infection since using silver gel.

Use with Other Supplements

Structured silver reduces the burden of bacteria, viruses and yeast. As a result, supplements that help stimulate the immune system will have a greater ability to work with an immune system that has a greater capacity to perform as it should.

Vaginal Cleanse (See Women's Issues)

Vaginal Odor

Vaginal odor can often be caused by a yeast or bacterial infection. Structured silver can be used as a douche by pumping two ounces of silver liquid intravaginally, holding it for 12 twelve minutes, and then rinsing. Apply silver gel to a tampon and insert into the vagina.

For continued problems, silver gel can be applied to the outer areas of the vaginal opening or placed on a panty liner.

Vaginitis

Vaginitis is term used for inflammation and irritation of the vagina caused by yeast or bacteria.

Symptoms of vaginitis include redness, inflammation, itching, burning, discomfort when urinating, possibly a foul vaginal odor, and sometimes an abnormal discharge or pain during intercourse.

Vaginitis is caused by a variety of yeast of bacteria, including Candida (yeast), Gardnerella (bacteria), Streptococcus (bacteria), Herpes (virus), and Trichomonas (parasite). Candida causes a watery, white, cottage cheese-like vaginal discharge that is irritating to the vagina and surrounding skin. Bacterial causes are usually associated with a fish-like odor and are associated with itching and irritation, but not during intercourse. Viruses can cause profuse discharge with a strong fish-like odor, pain upon urination, painful intercourse, and inflammation of the external genitals.

· Drink two teaspoons of silver liquid twice a day for one week or until symptoms subside.
· You can also apply silver gel topically to affected area twice a day. Or, apply the gel to tip of a tampon and insert into vagina for 90 minutes a day so the gel can stay in contact with germs in the vagina. Do this for one week.
· To create a structured silver douche, mix three ounces of silver liquid with three ounces of distilled water. Pump the solution into the vaginal cavity and hold for ten minutes, then release. This should be done once a day, for five days, or until symptoms are gone.
· Take at least 8 billion active culture probiotic daily. Reduce dietary sugar and carbohydrates. And take large quantities of antioxidants daily. This will help neutralize and clear free radicals produced by pathogens.

I have had several infections throughout my body, including yeast and bacterial infections. I tried structured silver and within 36 hours the yeast infection was gone. Within another 72 hours I had my blood tested again and found it to be bacteria-free. I've been taking the silver for three weeks and have not had a reoccurrence of any kind.

Structured silver can destroy bacteria, viruses, trichomonas and yeast in under ten minutes. This means you can expect the liquid and gel to destroy the cause of vaginitis as long as the structured silver stays in contact with the pathogen for ten minutes. The parasite trichomonas may take six weeks to eliminate. Most women feel noticeably better in one day and may return to normal in as little as two to five days.

Varicose Veins

Varicose or "spider" veins occur in the legs (and in the rectum as hemorrhoids). It causes the blood to have difficulty returning from the feet to the heart. Veins overstretch and bloat, causing a lot of pain. If the veins rupture, it's called an ulcer. Serious problems occur if these venostasis ulcers get infected.

Structured silver gel applied topically to the legs twice a day will help with pain and inflammation. Drinking structured silver liquid two teaspoons twice a day will allow the silver to circulate through the veins and arteries of the system.

Walking is essential to getting the blood flow moving again in varicose veins. I recommend stretching and walking 25 minutes each day.

Viral Infections (See antiviral)

Viruses

A virus is a sub-microscopic infectious agent that is unable to grow or reproduce outside a host cell. We generally fight viruses with antibiotics. However, antibiotics do not actually destroy the virus. For many viruses, such as influenza or the bird flu, there are virtually no beneficial drugs or treatment.

Structured silver resonates at a frequency that can actually suppress and contain viral infections by interfering with the duplication and replication of viral infections. If you can stop a virus from duplicating in the first four hours of infection, you have a good chance of stopping symptoms entirely.

When the herpes virus infects the skin, we call it a canker sore or cold sore. If you use structured silver within the first four hours of feeling the sore, it will not even erupt. However, if you don't get it in the early phases, viral infection will duplicate and become much more difficult to control. This is why regular, preventive use is so important.

To fight viruses, structured silver can be taken internally as a liquid, topically as a gel, or inhaled to combat sinus problems. You can expect a noticeable benefit to be felt within the first two hours and significant benefits within the first two days.

Vitamins, Minerals, Essential Fatty Acids, Amino acids

By combining structured silver liquid and gel with vitamins, minerals, essential fatty acids, and amino acids, you will boost immunity by reducing stress on the immune system.

Warts

Warts are usually viral infections that have gotten under the skin and reproduced in a way that makes thickened, callused tissue around it. If you can get the structured silver down inside the wart it will actually kill the virus and it will die. By drinking two teaspoons of structured silver twice a day, it will circulate in your bloodstream. Combined with topical application of the gel, you should see significant benefit.

For quicker, more complete results, pare down the wart with a sharp instrument. (Warts do not have pain receptors. When you feel pain, you've reached the skin). Put the structured silver on the exposed portion of the wart.

Water Purification

Water can be purified using silver liquid. By applying four drops of structured silver liquid into eight-ounce glass of water, and letting it stand for about two minutes, it will purify even raw river water. Add 32 ounces of liquid structured silver to a 55-gallon drum of water to keep your water storage purified for years.

The EPA reports that 40 percent of all water is unfit to drink. I have had the experience of drinking water in foreign countries and suffering the consequences. I've gotten food poisoning twice. The first time, I did not have structured silver liquid and it took me two weeks to get over my diarrhea. I learned my lesson. I took silver after the second occurrence and remedied the problem within two hours.

Wind Burn

A windburn dries out the skin. Structured silver gel with aloe is very effective as a skin moisturizer. For severely chapped and bleeding skin, structured silver gel with aloe can be mixed with Vaseline, in a 1:1 ratio. This will keep the skin very moist. After one application of this mixture, structured silver can be applied topically on its own, as needed, for up to two weeks.

Wipes

You can create your own structured silver disposable wipes. Simply put structured silver liquid on a small napkins and carry in a zip lock bag. These antibacterial wipes can be used to clean hands, remove makeup, clean wounds, or sanitize public surfaces.

Nearly 70 percent of all contagious diseases are transferred by hand contact. These wipes will greatly reduce the amount of germs that come in contact with your system.

Women's Issues

The fact that silver is antibacterial, antiviral and antifungal makes this unique liquid the perfect vaginal cleanse. It can be very difficult to identify the source of vaginal problems/diseases due to the fact that they could be bacterial, viral or fungal. Structured silver vaginal cleansing destroys all these sources of vaginal disease. For these and many more reasons structured silver can cleanse multiple sources of vaginal disease including antibiotic resistant bacteria, STDs, yeast and do so safely as a liquid or gel.

The need for improved vaginal hygiene is evident when you research the sexually transmitted diseases, yeast infections, and occurrence of viral infections that cause cancer of the uterus and cervix. Structured silver liquid destroys the cause of numerous vaginal diseases and will become a woman's best friend when it comes to itching, cramping and yeast infections.

For more detailed information, see the chapter entitled on women's health.

Wound Healing

Wounds come in many forms—burns, cuts, lacerations, bruises, broken bones. Structured silver has been documented to help improve wound healing. In a study done at the University of Utah, pigs healed substantially faster and had less bacteria, viruses, and mold when treated with structured silver.

Silver gel can be applied topically to any wound one to four times a day. By keeping the wound moist, it will improve quicker and with less scarring. Drinking two teaspoons of liquid structured silver twice a day will help improve wounds in the nose, ears, eyes, nose, throat, or any part of the body.

Yeast

Yeast can infect the vagina, cervix, uterus or vulvar opening, resulting in tissue damage of the affected areas.

Symptoms of a Candida yeast infection include redness, irritation, flaking skin, foul odor, itching, burning, and discomfort when urinating or during intercourse. May be associated with abnormal discharge. Usually causes a watery, white, cottage cheese-like vaginal discharge that is irritating to the vagina and surrounding skin.

- Drink two teaspoons of silver liquid twice a day for one week or until symptoms subside.
- You can also apply silver gel topically to affected area twice a day. Or, apply the gel to tip of a tampon and insert into vagina for 90 minutes a day so the gel can stay in contact with germs in the vagina. Do this for one week.
- To create a structured silver douche, mix three ounces of silver liquid with three ounces of distilled water. Pump the solution into the vaginal cavity and hold for ten minutes, then release. This should be done once a day, for five days, or until symptoms are gone.
- Take at least 8 billion active culture probiotic daily. Reduce dietary sugar and carbohydrates. And take large quantities of antioxidants daily. This will help neutralize and clear free radicals produced by pathogens.
- Capryllic acid has been shown to help reduce intestinal yeast and may help if the yeast is systemic.

Structured silver can destroy yeast in less than ten minutes. This means you can expect the liquid and gel to destroy the cause of yeast infections as long as the structured silver stays in contact with the pathogen for ten minutes. Most women feel noticeably better in one day and may return to normal in as little as two to five days.

Women's Health and Silver

This chapter collects information presented elsewhere in the hope that as many women as possible will take advantage of silver's amazing benefits for female health. Many women who struggle with vaginal infections simply suffer in silence after years of unsuccessful attempts to restore balance and health. Silver offers new hope and a tremendous track record for overcoming problems. After speaking with thousands of women before and after they began to use silver, I sincerely hope that this information will also be of service to you.

For vaginal infections, a general recommendation is helpful. I suggest consulting the following pages for greater detail, but here are some quick notes regarding vaginal use:

- To quickly control a vaginal infection, structured silver liquid can be used as a douche. Two ounces of the product can be pumped intravaginally, held for 12 minutes, and then released. Gel can then be applied to the surface.
- Structured silver can help prevent vaginal infections. By putting gel on a tampon before inserting, you will receive antibacterial, antiviral, anti-mold, and even anti-parasitic benefits. This method can be used for 30 minutes at a time, four hours apart.
- Liquid or gel can be used in a panty liner for an added layer of protection.
- In addition to keeping yeast and bacterial infections under control, when used as a personal lubricant on the surface of condoms, silver has the potential to kill viruses and sexually transmitted diseases.
- Silver can be used in the bathtub. Pour in four ounces and enjoy a warm bath for 25 minutes. This will cleanse the vagina and anus.

For topical and cosmetic applications, many women like to use gel, but the liquid can be applied topically as well. Purse-sized spray containers, cotton balls, gauze, and soaking are all easy ways to gain a topical benefit of silver using the liquid if a gel is unavailable. Both liquid and gel are great options for topical use.

1. Bacterial Infections of the Vagina (Vaginosis, Itching, Odor, etc.)

Description: A bacteria-caused infection of the vagina and vulva.

Symptoms: Redness, itching, inflammation, bumps, irritation, and burning when urinating. Usually causes a discharge with fishlike odor and is associated with itching and irritation.

Causes: Streptococcus, Garnerella, sexually transmitted diseases, lack of the female hormone estrogen, poor hygiene, and contamination from the rectum.

Recommendations:

- Silver liquid: Drink two tsps minimum twice a day for prevention and treatment.
- Silver gel: Apply to affected area two to five times a day for as long as needed.
- Silver gel applied to a tampon and inserted into the vagina for 90 minutes a day where the gel can stay in contact with the germs in the vagina.
- Silver douche: Use three ounces of structured silver liquid and mix it with three ounces of distilled water and pump the solution into the vaginal cavity and hold for ten minutes, then release. This should be done once a day, for five

days, or until symptoms are gone.

· Take daily probiotics (at least 8 billion active cultures) every day.
· Reduce dietary sugars and carbohydrates.
· By taking large doses of antioxidants you can expect to neutralize and clear the free radicals produced by the pathogens.

What you can expect: Silver have destroyed the bacteria that cause vaginosis in under six minutes of contact in numerous scientific studies. This means you can expect the liquid and gel to destroy the cause of vaginosis, as long as the silver stays in contact with the pathogen for six minutes. Most women feel noticeably better in one day and may return to normal in as little as two to five days.

2. Chlamydia (see also Contamination from Sex)

Description: Chlamydia is a type of bacteria that is transferred by sexual contact. It destroys the tissues inside the vagina and returns when the immune system is depressed. It is also called the clap.

Symptoms: Pain, inflammation, rash and tissue damage.

Cause: Bacteria inside vagina and surrounding area.

Recommendations:

· Silver liquid: Drink two teaspoons twice a day for prevention.
· Use silver gel with aloe as a personal lubricant, on the male and female genitals prior to sex. It is a water-soluble gel that lubricates just like K-Y Jelly. Silver gel can be effective against sexually transmitted diseases like gonorrhea, syphilis, AIDS, herpes simplex, and Chlamydia.
· Use silver gel on the condom to lubricate and destroy the bacteria, viruses, and yeast that may be transferred during intercourse.

3. Cramps (see also Painful Menstruation)

Description: Muscle cramps in vaginal wall and uterus.

Symptoms: Muscle cramps that result in pain and suffering.

Causes: Lack of oxygen in the muscles, muscle spasms, nerve irritation, and toxins in the bloodstream and muscles.

Recommendations:

· Silver liquid: Drink two tablespoons twice a day to help destroy the toxins in the bloodstream.
· Silver gel: Apply to the sore muscles twice daily.
· Take calcium and magnesium supplements.

4. Contamination from Sex

Description: Exchanging germs during intercourse.

Symptoms: Infections of the genitalia and surrounding area from bacteria, viruses, and yeast resulting tissue damage, itching, burning, and long-term chronic disease.

Cause: Bacteria, viruses, and yeast infecting the genitalia.

Recommendations:

· Silver liquid: Drink two teaspoons twice a day for prevention.
· Use silver gel as a personal lubricant, on the male and female genitals prior to sex. It is a water-soluble gel that lubricates just like K-Y Jelly. Structured silver gel can be effective against sexually transmitted diseases like gonorrhea, syphilis, HIV, herpes simplex, and chlamydia.
· Use silver gel on the condom to lubricate and destroy the bacteria, viruses, and yeast that may be transferred during intercourse.

5. Endometriosis (see Painful Menstruation)

Description: Severe uterine pain during menstruation.

Symptoms: The main symptom of endometriosis is pain concentrated in the lower abdomen and may localize to one side of the abdomen or radiate pain to the thighs and low back. Other symptoms include sharp, throbbing, dull, nauseating, burning, or shooting pains during dysmenorrheal (painful menstruation). Endometriosis may be present in the long or short term and may precede menstruation by several days or may accompany it and usually subsides as menstruation tapers off. This severe pain may coexist with excessively heavy blood loss. On rare occasions, nausea, vomiting, diarrhea, headache, dizziness, or disorientation may present.

Causes: Prostaglandins are inflammatory compounds that are released during menstruation and they cause the muscles of the uterus to contract. The uterus muscles constrict so much that the blood supply is compressed, reducing the delivery of blood to the sensitive tissues of the endometrium. The absence of blood flow to the endometrium causes pain and cramping as the tissues die from the lack of blood. The uterus begins to contract in such a strong manner that the dead tissues are squeezed out of the uterus and out through the cervix and vagina. This temporary oxygen deprivation in the uterus is responsible for the cramps and pain. Silver makes dramatic improvements in wound healing and pain management inside the uterus and reduces inflammation, which can help reduce the cause of this painful menstruation.

Recommendations:

· Silver liquid: take two tsps minimum twice a day for prevention and treatment.
· Silver gel applied topically to affected area of pain two to five times a day for as long as needed.
· Silver gel applied to a tampon and inserted into the vagina for 90 minutes a day where the gel can stay in contact with the wounds in the vagina.
· Silver douche: Use three ounces of structured silver liquid and mix it with three ounces of distilled water and pump the solution into the vaginal cavity and hold for ten minutes, then release. This should be done once a day, for five days, or until symptoms are gone.
· Optional uses: Pour four ounces of liquid silver into a warm full tub of water, then bathe, soak and relax, flushing the silver water into the vaginal cavity. Twenty-five minutes is average for a muscle-relaxing vaginal flush in the tub.

Additional Products: Herbal products that help reduce inflammation, pain, and hormone balance include, black cohosh, blue vervain, Suma, and white willow.

6. Gonorrhea (see also Contamination from Sex)

Recommendations:

· Silver liquid: Drink two teaspoons twice a day for prevention.
· Use structured silver gel as a personal lubricant, on the male and female genitals prior to sex. It is a water-soluble gel that lubricates just like K-Y Jelly. Structured silver gel can be effective against sexually transmitted diseases like gonorrhea, syphilis, AIDS, herpes simplex, and chlamydia.
· Use structured silver gel on the condom to lubricate and destroy the bacteria, viruses, and yeast that may be transferred during intercourse.

7a. Herpes Virus (see also Viral Vaginal Infections)

Description: Herpes virus infections within and outside the vagina.

Symptoms: Water blisters inside and outside the vagina producing extremely painful conditions depending on the severity of the lesions of blisters.

Causes: Herpes virus.

Recommendations:

- Silver liquid: swallow two teaspoons at minimum twice a day for prevention and treatment.
- Silver gel applied topically to affected area two to five times a day for as long as needed.
- Silver gel applied to a tampon and inserted into the vagina for 90 minutes a day where the gel can stay in contact with the germs in the vagina.
- Silver douche: Use three ounces of structured silver liquid and mix it with three ounces of distilled water and pump the solution into the vaginal cavity and hold for ten minutes, then release. This should be done once a day, for five days, or until symptoms are gone.
- Take daily probiotics (at least 8 billion active cultures) every day.
- Reduce dietary sugars and carbohydrates.
- By taking large doses of antioxidants you can expect to neutralize and clear the free radicals produced by the pathogens.

What you can expect: Silver can destroy the virus that causes infections in under six minutes. This means you can expect the liquid and gel to destroy the cause of viral infections as long as the silver stays in contact with the pathogen for six minutes. Most women feel noticeably better in one day and may return to normal in as little as two to five days.

7b. Herpes Simplex (Fever Blisters)

Recommendations:

- Silver liquid: swallow two teaspoons at minimum twice a day for prevention and treatment.
- Silver gel applied topically to affected area two to five times a day for as long as needed.

· The sooner the gel gets on the blister the faster it will heal. If you get the gel on the wound (and keep it moist with gel) in the first four hours that the blister erupts it will stop it from erupting and shrink back to normal without rupturing or spreading. The key is to get silver gel on the wound as soon as you feel a punch or sting and keep the gel on every 30 minutes for the first four hours.

8. Hysterectomy / Pelvic Inflammatory Disease

Description: Chronic inflammation of the pelvic region due to ongoing infections.

Symptoms: Long-term inflammation and infections of the vagina, vulva, uterus, and surrounding tissues. It may be painful for a short or long period of time and is aggravated by urination, sexual activity or yeast overgrowth.

Symptoms: Extreme pain, inflammation, and possible nausea, with fever.

Causes: Bacteria, viruses, and yeast.

Recommendations:

· Silver liquid: Drink two teaspoons twice a day for prevention or drink two tablespoons twice a day for severe conditions.
· Silver gel: Apply to the affected and painful area at least twice a day to destroy the pathogens that cause the pain and infection.
· Silver douche: Use three ounces of structured silver liquid and mix it with three ounces of distilled water and pump the solution into the vaginal cavity and hold for ten minutes, then release. This should be done once a day, for five days, or until symptoms are gone.
· Optional uses: Pour four ounces of liquid silver into a warm full tub of water, then bathe, soak, and relax, flushing the silver water into the vaginal cavity. Twenty-five minutes is average for a muscle relaxing vaginal flush in the tub.

9. Human Papillomavirus (HPV) (see also Viral Vaginal Infections)

Description: A viral infection usually afflicting the cervix where it destroys the cellular structure of the cells and can damage the DNA, causing cancer of the cervix.

Symptoms: Most of the time there are no symptoms except lab tests performed by the doctor. There is no real treatment from the doctor until the tissue damage by the virus has become cancerous. At this point surgery is performed. Structured silver liquid douche and gel on a tampon can give the woman a method of destroying the cause of the abnormal cells and possible prevention of the cause of the cancer.

Cause: Human Papillomavirus (HPV)

Recommendations:

- Silver liquid: swallow two teaspoons at minimum twice a day for prevention and treatment.
- Silver gel applied to the tip of a tampon and inserted into the vagina for 90 minutes a day where the gel can stay in contact with the germs in the vagina against the cervix.
- Silver douche: Use three ounces of structured silver liquid and mix it with three ounces of distilled water and pump the solution into the vaginal cavity and hold for ten minutes, then release. This should be done once a day, for five days, or until symptoms are gone.
- Take daily probiotics (at least 8 billion active cultures) every day.
- Reduce dietary sugars and carbohydrates.
- By taking large doses of antioxidants you can expect to neutralize and clear the free radicals produced by the pathogens.

What you can expect: Silver can destroy the virus's ability to replicate, reducing the level of viral infection over time. Silver can inhibit the replication of both types of viral replication (RNA and DNA). Most women feel noticeably better in one day and may return to normal in as little as two to five days.

10. Infertility

Description: Inability to get pregnant or carry a pregnancy to full term.

Causes: Approximately 10% of couples have difficulty conceiving and 25% of the time it is the male that is infertile. Genetic factors, diabetes reduces blood flow, pituitary, hypothalamus, pituitary problems reduce fertility.

In addition, the following toxins have been shown to cause infertility: glues, volatile solvents, silicones, pesticides, and chemical dusts. Tobacco smokers are 60% more likely to be infertile because smoking increases the chances of miscarriage by 30%. Infections of the blood, vagina, cervix, vulva or male organs can contribute to reproductive organ infections, which interfere with fertility. (Silver can reduce this problem by destroying bacteria, viruses, and fungus that cause the infections, including sexually transmitted diseases). It has been reported that an adenovirus reduces fertility and it should be noted that silver destroys this type of virus.

Recommendations:

- Silver liquid: two teaspoons at minimum twice a day.
- Silver gel used during intercourse to prevent sexually transmitted diseases, yeast infections, and bacterial vaginosis.
- Silver gel applied to vaginal opening and male genitals daily to reduce pathogens.
- Remember that silver will destroy the bacteria, viruses, and yeast if it stays in contact with the germ for six to ten minutes.
- Follow your doctor's recommendations concerning ovulation, supplements, stimulants, hormones etc.

11. Menopause

Description: Hormone changes that produce physiologic, behavioral and mental changes.

Symptoms: Mental anxiety, delusion, hot flashes, pain, cessation of menstruation, aging, and skin degeneration.

Causes: Reduction in the female hormones resulting in changes in the normal physiologic functions, mental wellbeing, and behavioral adjustments to the changes in hormones.

Sometimes bacteria or fungus can negatively affect the hormone balance from the ovaries. With the changes in hormone levels the skin loses some of its ability to maintain flexible, regenerative abilities.

Recommendations for Skin During Menopause:

- Silver liquid: Drink two teaspoons at minimum twice a day to prevent and maintain wellness.
- Silver gel applied to the face, head, neck, and all other skin areas to help reduce bacterial, viral, and fungal infections. The gel helps with existing wounds and long-term scars. Apply to these wounds or scars twice daily for three months and expect significant improvement in wound healing and reduction of existing scars, while preventing the cause of acne and premature aging.

12. Painful Menstruation, Dysmenorrhea, Menstrual Cramps, Endometriosis, and PMS

Description: Severe uterine pain during menstruation.

Symptoms: The main symptom of dysmenorrheal is pain concentrated in the lower abdomen and may localize to one side of the abdomen or radiate pain to the thighs and lower back. Other symptoms include sharp, throbbing, dull, nauseating, burning, or shooting pains are noted during dysmenorrheal (painful menstruation). Dysmenorrhea may precede menstruation by several days or may accompany it and usually subsides as menstruation tapes off. This severe pain may coexist with excessively heavy blood loss. On rare occasions, nausea, vomiting, diarrhea, headache, dizziness, or disorientation may present.

Causes: Prostaglandins are inflammatory compounds that are released during menstruation and they cause the muscles of the uterus to contract. The uterus muscles constrict so much that the blood supply is compressed, reducing the delivery of blood to the sensitive tissues of the endometrium. The absence of blood flow to the endometrium causes pain and cramping as the tissues die from the lack of blood. The uterus begins to contract in such a strong manner that the dead tissues are squeezed out of the uterus and out through the cervix and vagina. This temporary oxygen deprivation in the uterus is responsible for the cramps and pain. Silver makes dramatic improvements in wound healing and pain management inside the uterus and reduces inflammation, which can help reduce the cause of this painful menstruation.

Recommendations:

- Silver liquid: swallow two teaspoons at minimum twice a day for prevention and treatment.
- Silver gel applied topically to affected area two to five times a day for as long as needed.
- Silver gel applied to a tampon and inserted into the vagina for 90 minutes a day where the gel can stay in contact with the wounds in the vagina.
- Silver douche: Use three ounces of structured silver liquid and mix it with three ounces of distilled water and pump the solution into the vaginal cavity and hold for ten minutes, then release. This should be done once a day, for five days, or until symptoms are gone.
- Optional uses: Pour four ounces of liquid silver into a warm full tub of water, then bathe, soak, and relax, flushing the silver water into the vaginal cavity. Twenty-five minutes is average for a muscle relaxing vaginal flush in the tub.

Additional Products: Herbal products that help reduce inflammation, pain, and hormone balance include, black cohosh, blue vervain, Suma, and white willow.

13. Pre Menstrual Syndrome (PMS) (see Painful Menstruation)

14. Sexually Transmitted Diseases (see also Contamination from Sex)

Recommendations:

- Silver liquid: Drink two teaspoons at minimum twice a day for prevention.
- Use structured silver gel as a personal lubricant, on the male and female genitals prior to sex. It is a water-soluble gel that lubricates just like K-Y Jelly. Structured silver gel can be effective against sexually transmitted diseases like gonorrhea, syphilis, AIDS, herpes simplex, and chlamydia.
- Use silver gel on the condom to lubricate and destroy the bacteria, viruses, and yeast that may be transferred during intercourse.

15. Skin Infections, Acne, and Mastitis

Description: Infections in and under the skin.

Symptoms: Infections under the skin, causing the inflammation and the destruction of healthy skin tissues resulting in pustules, cysts, boils, and inflamed painful tissues.

Causes: Bacteria, viruses, and fungus that infects healthy skin topically and under the surface of the skin.

Recommendations:

- Silver liquid: Drink two teaspoons at minimum twice a day for wellness.
- Silver gel: Apply to infected areas at least twice a day (up to six times a day) to destroy the cause of the infection. Alternately, a small spray bottle, easily carried in a purse or backpack, can be used on the skin throughout the day.
- For the face: Apply structured silver gel as soon as you leave the shower and have pat dried the face. Then wait two minutes for the gel to penetrate the skin after which you can apply makeup.
- For other skin infections like mastitis or athletes foot: Apply the gel to the skin twice a day or more as needed.

· If the gel can penetrate the skin and get the source of the infection, it can kill the bacteria in six minutes.

16. Syphilis (see also Contamination from Sex)

Recommendations:

· Silver liquid: Drink two teaspoons at minimum twice a day for prevention.
· Use structured silver gel as a personal lubricant, on the male and female genitals prior to sex. It is a water-soluble gel that lubricates just like K-Y Jelly. Silver gel will destroy the sexually transmitted diseases like gonorrhea, syphilis, aids, herpes simplex, and chlamydia.
· Use structured silver gel on the condom to lubricate and destroy the bacteria, viruses, and yeast that may be transferred during intercourse.

17. Urinary Tract Infection (UTI)

Description: A urinary infection (UTI) is bacterial infection that affects any part of the urinary tract. The kidney, ureters, and bladder are adversely affected by invading bacteria that multiply in the urine.

Symptoms: The most common symptom is pain and burning during urination, more frequent urination, an abnormal urgency to urinate without vaginal discharge.

A kidney infection may present with pain in the lower back or flank area with possible more serious symptoms of chills nausea, vomiting, and high fever.

A bladder infection (called cystitis) is usually associated with abdominal pain, incontinence, blood in urine, pus in urine, inability to urinate despite the urge, and malaise.

Causes: Bacteria, viruses, and fungus that infect the genital area.

Recommendations:

· Silver liquid: Drink two ounces every hour for four hours. Since silver destroys the bacteria that cause the infection in six minutes, it is important to absorb large amounts of silver for four hours. In this way the silver can wash through the kidneys and pool in the bladder. Silver passes through the body unchanged, meaning that the silver that pools in the bladder will still kill the bacteria in the kidneys, bladder, and urethra.

- Silver gel: Apply topically twice a day to affected area twice a day or as needed.
- Take 8 billion active cultures of Probiotics containing acidophilus and bifidus daily.
- By taking large doses of antioxidants you can expect to neutralize and clear the free radicals produced by the pathogens.
- Cranberry is terrific at helping reduce bladder infections.

What you can expect: Silver can destroy the bacteria that cause infections in the urinary tract in under six minutes. This means you can expect the liquid and gel to destroy the cause of the UTI as long as the silver stays in contact with the pathogen for six minutes. Most women feel noticeably better in two hours and may return to normal in as little as four to six hours.

18. Vaginitis

Description: Inflammation and irritation of the vagina caused by yeast or bacteria causing pain, itching, and discomfort in the vaginal area.

Symptoms: It can produce redness, inflammation, itching, burning, discomfort when urinating, possibly a foul vaginal odor, and may be associated with abnormal discharge or pain during intercourse. Additional notes:

- Candida causes watery, white, cottage-cheese-like vaginal discharge, which is irritating to the vagina and the surrounding skin.
- Bacterial causes are usually associated with a fishlike odor and is associated with itching and irritation but not during intercourse.
- Viruses can cause profuse discharge with a strong fishlike odor, pain upon urination, painful intercourse, and inflammation of the external genitals.

Causes: Candida (yeast), Gardnerella (bacteria), Streptococcus (bacteria), Herpes (virus), Trichomonas (parasite).

Recommendations:

- Silver liquid: Drink two teaspoons at minimum twice a day for one week or until symptoms subside.
- Silver gel: Apply topically twice a day to affected area and apply structured silver gel to the tip of a tampon and insert into the vagina for 90 minutes a day for a week.
- Silver douche: Use three ounces of structured silver liquid and mix it with

three ounces of distilled water and pump the solution into the vaginal cavity and hold for ten minutes, then release. This should be done once per day for five days or until symptoms are gone.

· Stop eating sugars, yeasts, and breads that feed the yeast.
· Take 8 billion active cultures of Probiotics that contain acidophilus and bifidus daily.
· By taking large doses of antioxidants you can expect to neutralize and clear the free radicals produced by the pathogens.

What you can expect: structured silver can destroy bacteria, viruses and yeast in under ten minutes. This means you can expect the liquid and gel to destroy the cause of vaginitis as long as the structured silver stays in contact with the pathogen for ten minutes. The parasite trichomonas may take six weeks to completely eliminate. Most women feel noticeably better in one day and may return to normal in as little as two to five days.

19. Vaginal Bleeding (see also Painful Menstruation)

Recommendations:

· Silver gel applied topically to affected area two to five times a day for as long as needed.
· Silver gel applied to a tampon and inserted into the vagina for 90 minutes a day where the gel can stay in contact with the wounds in the vagina.
· Silver douche: Use three ounces of structured silver liquid and mix it with three ounces of distilled water and pump the solution into the vaginal cavity and hold for ten minutes, then release. This should be done once a day, for five days, or until symptoms are gone.
· Silver liquid: swallow two teaspoons at minimum twice a day for prevention and treatment.
· Optional uses: Pour four ounces of liquid silver into a warm full tub of water, then bathe, soak, and relax, flushing the silver water into the vaginal cavity. Twenty-five minutes is average for a muscle relaxing vaginal flush in the tub.

Additional Products: Herbal products that help reduce inflammation, pain, and hormone balance include, black cohosh, blue vervain, Suma, and white willow.

20. Vaginal Dryness

Recommendations:

- Silver gel should be applied twice a day or as many times as needed to lubricate the vulva and vagina and to help prevent infections, inflammation, and disease.
- Silver gel can be applied to the penis, vulva, and vagina or on the condom to help lubricate during intercourse. Apply liberally, knowing that it does not contain any alcohol (so it won't irritate the sensitive tissues of the vagina) and it does not contain any petroleum (so it will not cause stickiness, greasiness or macerate the vulva).

21. Vaginal Infections, Trichomoniasis, Chlamydia, Viral Vaginitis Vulvitis, and Vulvodynia (see also UTI)

Recommendations:

- Silver liquid: Drink two teaspoons at minimum twice a day for prevention.
- Use silver gel as a personal lubricant, on the male and female genitals prior to sex. It is a water-soluble gel that lubricates just like K-Y Jelly. Silver gel can be effective against sexually transmitted diseases like gonorrhea, syphilis, AIDS, herpes simplex, and chlamydia.
- Use structured silver gel on the condom to lubricate and destroy the bacteria, viruses, and yeast that may be transferred during intercourse.

22. Viral Vaginal Infections

Description: Viruses like herpes that reside in the vaginal cavity and surrounding skin, cervix, and uterus.

Symptoms: Water blisters on the genital region, about one week after infection, associated with tenderness, swollen glands, and fever. The water blisters are extremely painful and heal in about three weeks unless silver is used where prevention is possible and wound healing is as much as three times faster (one week).

Causes: Viruses (herpes, etc.).

Recommendations:

- Silver liquid: swallow two teaspoons at minimum twice a day for prevention and treatment.

- Silver gel applied topically to affected area two to five times a day for as long as needed.
- Silver gel applied to a tampon and inserted into the vagina for 90 minutes a day where the gel can stay in contact with the germs in the vagina.
- Silver douche: Use three ounces of structured silver liquid and mix it with three ounces of distilled water and pump the solution into the vaginal cavity and hold for ten minutes, then release. This should be done once a day, for five days, or until symptoms are gone.
- Take daily probiotics (at least 8 billion active cultures) every day.
- Reduce dietary sugars and carbohydrates.
- By taking large doses of antioxidants you can expect to neutralize and clear the free radicals produced by the pathogens.

What you can expect: Silver can inhibit the replication of viruses, resulting in a gradual reduction in the viral load. Most women feel noticeably better in one day and may return to normal in as little as two to five days.

23. Yeast Infections (Candida)

Description: Yeast that has infected the vagina, cervix, uterus, or vulvar opening, resulting in tissue damage on the affected areas.

Symptoms: Redness, irritation, flaking skin, foul odor, itching, burning, and/or discomfort when urinating or during intercourse. May be associated with abnormal discharge. Usually causes a watery, white, cottage-cheese-like vaginal discharge, which is irritating to the vagina and surrounding skin.

Causes: Yeast (Candida).

Recommendations:

- Silver liquid: Drink two teaspoons at minimum twice a day for one week or until symptoms subside
- Silver gel: Apply topically twice a day to affected area and apply structured silver gel to the tip of a tampon and insert into the vagina for 90 minutes a day for a week.
- Silver douche: Use three ounces of structured silver liquid and mix it with three ounces of distilled water and pump the solution into the vaginal cavity

and hold for ten minutes, then release. This should be done once a day, for five days, or until symptoms are gone.

· Stop eating sugars, yeasts, and breads that feed the yeast.
· Take 8 billion active cultures of Probiotics that contain acidophilus and bifidus daily.
· By taking large doses of antioxidants you can expect to neutralize and clear the free radicals produced by the pathogens.
· Capryllic acid has been shown to help reduce intestinal yeast and may help if the yeast is systemic.

What you can expect: Silver can destroy yeast in under ten minutes. This means you can expect the liquid and gel to destroy the cause of yeast infections as long as the silver stays in contact with the pathogen for ten minutes. Most women feel noticeably better in one day and may return to normal in as little as two to five days.

24. Wellness

Description: The habits that promote constant wellness and disease-free living, which promotes a wholeness and foundation for happy living.

Symptoms: Healthy body systems, normal constant wellness, balanced and self-reliant immunity, and the ability to defend against environmental pathogens.

Causes: The cause of wellness is an attitude, combined with healthy genetics, and supported with eating correctly, sleeping sufficiently to recharge, exercise, regular cleansing, reduction of stress, and supplementing where there are deficiencies or greater needs. Silver is the perfect supplement for healthy living because it destroys the cause of most disease-causing bacteria, viruses, and yeast. Taking silver daily reduces the workload on an already overworked immune system. Silver can be your first line of defense because it supports a healthy immune system and works directly on any part of the body that is infected, weakened or in need of healing. By taking silver two teaspoons twice a day you are promoting wellness. In the event you need to use more, it is safe to double or quadruple the amount for up to a month. The gel is magnificent because it works wherever you apply it, inside or outside the body.

Recommendations:

· Silver liquid: Drink two teaspoons twice a day for prevention and double it when there is more demand.

- Silver gel: Apply to wounds, scratches, scrapes, vaginal infections, mouth, nose, throat or wherever there is need to destroy germs. The gel can be safely used as much as one to ten times a day for three months at a time, then return to normal or near-normal usage.

Animals: Cats, Dogs and Horses

Animals and humans have similar health needs. Millions of people consider their pets to be part of the family. For that reason, pet health is a major concern. While there are specialized health care options for animals ranging from advanced surgical procedures to any number of pharmaceutical drugs, there is also a natural solution for a broad array of pet health needs. This solution is a pH–balanced structured silver.

Animals in General

- Wash wounds with silver liquid
- Apply silver gel to the wound and surrounding areas (this should be done 1-4 times a day as needed)
- Wraps can be used to keep the gel in place longer
- Animals can drink the liquid silver for system benefits. It is given in amounts proportionate to the body weight of the animal. The average human weighs 150 pounds and drinks 2 teaspoons twice a day (maintenance dose). Animals receive a dose of silver liquid that is based on the weight of the animal in comparison to human doses.

Example:
Human weight 150 pounds: dose of two teaspoons a day
Animal weight 15 pounds: dose of one tenth as much twice a day
(usually a dose of ½ teaspoon twice a day is the smallest dose given)
Animal weight 1500 pounds: dose of ten times as much twice a day
(usually a dose of 4 ounces given twice a day is the largest dose given)

- For more serious conditions the dose can be doubled, tripled or even quadrupled.
- Gel can be given topically, orally and/or in every orifice of the body in doses that cover the wound or treat the orifice, usually twice a day, but it is safe enough to apply 5 or more times a day (which is rarely needed).

For wounds in animals, it is recommended that the silver liquid and gel be given 60 days after total wound healing has been achieved to minimize scarring.

The point of using silver liquid and gel is that the silver will destroy the bacteria, viruses, yeast and numerous parasites if the silver can stay in contact with the pathogen for 6 minutes. When you apply the gel it is because it will stay in place longer than the liquid silver. Both can completely kill the pathogen but because the liquid silver is water-soluble it doesn't pass through the skin or other fatty tissues easily. In fact, it is because it cannot pass through lipids that it doesn't kill the good probiotic bacteria in the gut: the lactobacillus is coated with a milk fat that prevents water-soluble silver penetration and spares the good bacteria.

Silver liquid or gel can be added to drinking water, pumped into the mouth of the animal, applied to any orifice, and is actually absorbed very well rectally and vaginally.

12 Reasons to Use Alkaline Structured Silver for Your Pet

1. Protects against pathogens: Silver has been shown to effectively eradicate a number of bacteria, viruses, and other microbes, many of which are found in animals.
2. Supports the immune system.
3. Reduces inflammation: Through its disinfectant power, alkaline structured silver can reduce infection and slow the inflammatory response in animals.
4. Protects against many parasites.
5. Provides pain relief: Alkaline structured silver effectively reduces swelling and infection, and therefore reduces the associated pain without the side effects of traditional medicines.
6. Promotes oral health: Alkaline structured silver can help reduce tooth plaque and decay, and minimize bad breath. It also is effective for mouth and jaw infections.
7. Supports eye, ear and nose health: Alkaline structured silver is commonly applied to the eyes, ears, and nose for infections and other problems.
8. Keeps skin and coats healthy: Alkaline structured silver can effectively fight skin infections and help maintain a healthy coat.
9. Soothes wounds and burns: Can effectively heal wounds, scrapes, tears and burns.
10. Calms digestive ailments: Alkaline structured silver can safely be consumed to help with ailments of the digestive tract, such as food poisoning, vomiting, diarrhea and intestinal infections.
11. Disinfects pet surroundings: Alkaline structured silver is a terrific tool for disinfecting and cleaning your pet's surroundings, including dog and cat houses, litter boxes, food and water bowls, bird cages and so forth.

12. It is extremely SAFE: Dozens of studies, as well as thousands of anecdotal cases, have shown silver to be non-toxic and very safe for internal and external application.

Wound Protocols for Silver Liquid and Gel in Humans and Animals

My background includes specialization in the field of wound care, where I have given many presentations and have certification as a Fellow of the Academy of Professional Wound Care Association (FAPWCA). In my work in the field and with wounded U.S. Military personnel, I have seen some truly remarkable outcomes with silver and wounds.

This chapter describes silver application protocols for many common wounds.

1. MRSA and Serious Wound Infections

Causes: Methycillin Resistant Staphylococcus Aureus (MRSA). The bacteria is resistant to antibiotics and can consume healthy tissue including the skin, lungs, and vital organs. These infections can last for years or cause death in a day. There are approximately 30,000 new MRSA infections every day in America; one-fourth of these result in hospitalization. The cost to hospitals for the year 2008 was $30.5 billion just for treating this secondary infection usually acquired while residing in the hospital.

Silver Protocol For Minor MRSA Wounds:

- Drink 2 tablespoons of liquid silver (10 ppm or 30 ppm) per day.
- Wash wound with liquid silver once a day or as needed.
- Apply silver gel 2-3 times a day, until wound is healed and then for another 60 days to minimize scarring.
- Remember to use gel on hands and in nostrils to prevent systemic infections.

Silver Protocol For Serious MRSA Wounds:

- Drink 4 ounces a day (in divided doses, for 2 - 6 weeks or as needed).
- Apply silver gel twice daily or as needed up to ten times a day topically (for as long as needed to heal wound then apply gel once a day for 60 days to minimize scarring).

Surgical Debridement:

Clean wound and apply gel, with radical surgical excision often necessary. Hyperbaric oxygen therapy has been used empirically and can be used in conjunction with the administration of antibiotics, silver and surgical debridement.

Drug Treatments:

· Penicillin, 2 million units every 3 hours intravenously. (Other agents may include tetracycline, clindamycin, metronidazole, chloramphenicol, ceftoxitin)
· Silver liquid and or gel can be combined with antibiotic therapy resulting in synergistic benefits.

What You Can Expect: Wounds to heal three times faster than if they did not receive silver. Research shows this is due to the fact that there is less infection, inflammation and improved activation of stem cells.

NOTE: In general, silver liquid is used for prevention and treatment of minor wounds by drinking two teaspoons twice a day and applying the silver gel on the affected wound area, to the hands and in nostrils twice a day.

Infected wounds benefit from silver, which should be taken two tablespoons twice a day and the gel is applied to the affected wound area, the hands and nostrils twice a day.

In serious wounds, burns, infections, surgical injuries where there is significant tissue damage, silver liquid is swallowed 4 oz to 8 oz a day (in divided doses). The gel is applied to the wound and surrounding areas twice a day or as needed 1-10 times a day.

Silver gel and liquid can be used in every orifice of the body. Silver liquid and gel can be used in combination with antibiotics. But it is wise to take the silver one hour separate from the prescription drugs.

Structured pH-balanced (alkaline) silvers do not kill all the healthy probiotic bacteria in the gut, nor does it cause bacterial resistance. For this and other reasons structured pH balanced silvers can be used every day, for long periods of time, even if given in large doses for serious infections.

2. Post-Surgical Wounds

Causes: After surgery, injury or trauma that requires sutures or wound treatment.

Silver Protocol:

- Drink 2 tsps of liquid silver (10 ppm – 30 ppm) twice a day until wound heals.
- Apply silver gel twice daily to wound for one month after total healing to minimize scarring, remember to use gel on hands and in nostrils twice a day or as needed to prevent systemic infections.

Drug Treatment: Antibiotics as needed to prevent infection with options of anti-inflammatory and pain-killing prescriptions.

What You Can Expect: The average wound should heal twice to three times faster than the same wound would take to heal if there were no structured silver (as measured by time to wound closure, inflammation and infection). It is possible that you should expect to see noticeable benefits to the wound within the first day with measurable effects within one week (65% healed) and total healing in the most serious MRSA wounds within 5 weeks. Minor wounds, cuts, bites and other lacerations should heal three times faster.

3. Open Wounds

Causes: Trauma, injuries, compound fractures, rashes, infections, skin tears and skin ulcers.

Silver Protocol:

- Drink 2 teaspoons of liquid silver (10– 30 ppm) twice a day until wound heals.
- Apply silver gel to clean wound 1-3 times a day until wound completely heals, and then for one additional month to minimize scarring. Remember to use gel on hands and in nostrils to prevent systemic infections.

Drug Treatment: Antibiotics as needed to prevent infection with options of anti-inflammatory and pain-killing prescriptions.

In Immune Compromised and Drug Users: Drink 2 tablespoons of silver liquid 2-4 times a day and apply gel twice a day for one month after total healing has occurred. Remember to use gel on hands and in nostrils to prevent systemic infections.

What You Can Expect: Wounds heal three times faster than if they do not receive silver. This is due to the fact that there is less infection, inflammation and activation of stem cells.

4. Minor Wounds, Cuts, Lacerations, Scratches, Abrasions

Causes: Injuries, trauma, infections, surgery, bacteria, yeast.

Silver Protocol:

- Drink 2 teaspoons of liquid silver (10 – 30 ppm) twice a day until wound heals.
- Apply silver gel to clean wound 1-3 times a day until wound completely heals, and then for one additional month to minimize scarring.
- Remember to use gel on hands and in nostrils to prevent systemic infections.

Drug Treatment: Antibiotics as needed to prevent infection with options of anti-inflammatory and pain-killing prescriptions.

What You Can Expect: Wounds generally heal two to three times faster than a similar wound not receiving silver. You can expect mild and moderate pain relief within 10 minutes of application of the gel.

5. Skin Ulcers, Diabetic Ulcers, Bed Sores

Causes: Pressure, trauma, chronic injuries, diabetes, poor circulation, varicose veins.

Silver Protocol:

- Drink 2 tsps of liquid silver (10 ppm or 30 ppm) twice a day until wound heals.
- Apply silver gel to clean wound 1-3 times a day until wound completely heals, and then for one additional month to minimize scarring.
- Remember to use gel on hands and in nostrils to prevent systemic infections.

Drug Treatment:

- Antibiotics and diabetic medications as needed to prevent infection.
- Silver can be used together with prescription drug use resulting in a synergistic effect against infections.

What You Can Expect: You can expect less inflammation within one day. Infections take longer to heal but you should see improvements in the overall closure of the wound.

6. Bites (Animal and Human)

Causes: There are 900 dog bites a day in America requiring emergency room care. Cat bites are more likely to become infected, resulting in approximately 40% of all cat bites becoming infected. Human bites on humans become infected about 20% of the time. Cat, dog and other animal bites are polymicrobial, meaning they have numerous types of bacteria causing the infection. Pasturella species are the most common cause of dog and cat bites with others being staphylococcus, streptococcus and neisseria. Human bites average three aerobes and one anaerobe. These are the most common pathogens but many others have been found including stubborn strains of pseudomonas, staph MRSA, Haemophilus, and Eikenella corodens.

The reason a bite is so serious is because there is almost always a combination of pathogens. Antibiotics are effective on a narrow range of germs, while structured alkaline silver can destroy almost all the different pathogens.

Silver Protocol:

- Drink 2 tablespoons of liquid silver, twice a day. And continue for two weeks after total healing of the wound.
- If a serious infection occurs drink two ounces per day (in divided doses) until healed, and 30 days after total healing has occurred to minimize scarring.
- Wash wound area with silver liquid and apply silver gel twice a day for two weeks after total healing of the wound. Silver gel could be applied to the wound including the sutures and surrounding area.
- Studies demonstrate the importance of using silver gel on hands and in nostrils to prevent systemic infections in patients and health care professionals.
- Note silver can be combined with antibiotic therapy where it enhances the activity as much as tenfold (SOHO, 2006).

Drug Treatment:

For Bites that Need a Preventive Antibiotic: Use the following in combination with silver liquid and gel:

- For cat bites take dicloxacillin, 0.5 g orally four times a day for 3-5 days.
- This is a narrow spectrum of activity and I recommend using a broader-spectrum antibiotic, like cefuroxime, amoxicillin–clavulanic acid for prevention.

For Use in Infected Wounds: Use the following antibiotics in combination with silver gel and liquid:

- In general pasturella can be treated with penicillin or a tetracycline. Other more serious infections require second- and third-generation cephalosporins, fluoroquinolones or azithromycin and clarithromycin.
- Response is slow and therapy should be continued for at least 2-3 weeks.
- Human bites frequently require intravenous therapy with a beta lactam plus

beta lactmase inhibitor (unasyn, timentin, zosyn). And a second-generation cephalosporin with anaerobic activity (cefoxitin, cefotetan, cefetazole).

7. Burn Injuries

Causes: Heat, electrical, chemical, radiation, etc.

Silver Protocol:

- Drink two teaspoons liquid silver twice a day for minor burns (5 days) and apply silver gel twice a day or as needed.
- For more serious wounds drink two ounces a day (in divided doses) and apply gel 2-4 times a day. This should be applied for one month after the wound heals to minimize scarring.
- Another option is to apply silver gel to the bandage then place the silver gel on the wound, this will help keep it from being disturbed and reduce scarring and pain. It is possible to spray the liquid on the wound, spraying twice a day until wound heals.
- Remember to use gel on hands and in nostrils to prevent systemic infections.

Drug Treatment: Antibiotics and IV fluids can be prescribed in combination with silver liquid or gel, if necessary, to prevent and treat dehydration, pseudomonas and MRSA.

What You Can Expect: You can expect to reduce or eliminate infections, inflammation and promote stem cell activity. Burns heal faster than without silver, and you can expect reduction of minor and moderate pain within ten minutes of application. Structured silver should be used once daily for two months after the wound has healed to prevent abnormally large or striated scars. By doing this you should expect to have scars half the size of similar type wounds not being treated with structured alkaline silver.

8. Clostridial Myonecrosis (Gas Gangrene)

Causes: Trauma and injection drug use. Gangrene is caused by any of several clostridia: Clostridium perfrinigens, Clostridia ramosum, Clostridium bifermentuans, Clostridium histolyticusm, Clostridium novyi, etc.

Silver Protocol:

- Drink 2 table spoons of liquid silver per day.
- Wash wound with liquid silver once a day.
- Apply silver gel 2-3 times a day, until wound is healed and then for another 60 days.
- Remember to use gel on hands and in nostrils to prevent systemic infections.

Surgical Debridement: Exposure of infected areas are essential, with radical surgical excision often necessary. Hyperbaric oxygen therapy has been used empirically and can be used in conjunction with administration of antibiotic and surgical debridement.

Drug Treatments: Penicillin, 2 million units every 3 hours intravenously (other agents may include tetracycline, clindamycin, metronidazole, chloramphenicol, ceftoxitin). Silver liquid can be combined with antibiotic therapy, resulting in synergistic benefits (SOHO, 2006).

What You Can Expect: Reduction of infection is noticeable within twelve hours, with significant wound healing in one to three weeks. You can expect a reduced scar (50%) if you continue to apply the gel for two months after wound is healed.

9. Tetanus

Causes: Tetanus is caused by the neurotoxin tetanospasmin (Clostridium tetani). Spores of this organism are ubiquitous in soil and may germinate in a wound. Tetanospasmin interferes with neurotransmitters function at spinal synapses of inhibitory neurons, resulting in uncontrolled muscle spasms.

Silver Protocol:

- Drink 2 tablespoons of liquid silver (10 ppm or 30 ppm) per day.
- Wash wound with liquid silver once a day.
- Apply gel 2-3 times a day.
- Continue until wound is healed (about 2 weeks).
- Remember to use gel on hands and in nostrils to prevent systemic infections.

Drug Treatment: Prevention with vaccination is advised. Tetanus immune globulin 5000 units administered intramuscularly combined with bed rest (under the quietest conditions possible). Options include sedation and mechanical ventilation if required.

What You Can Expect: Helps with the drugs to promote synergistic healing. Each wound is different so healing times will differ but synergism with drugs and silver produce wound healing results quicker than individual treatments.

Frequently Asked Questions About Structured Silver

These questions have been asked thousands of times by newcomers to silver supplementation. For your convenience, here are simple answers:

Q: Why have liquid and gel?

A: The liquid can be used in all internal and topical applications. Some people prefer the gel for topical application. The gel is made of water, silver, and a gelling agent, whereas the liquid is made of only water and silver.

Q: What's up with the ppm (parts per million)?

A: What is essential to note is that "more ppm" does not equate to "stronger or better structured silver." 30 ppm doesn't kill better but it does kill some pathogens faster. If structured silver worked by chemical action or molar math alone, like a silver colloid product, higher concentrations would be important. But since structured silver works on pathogens through several mechanisms of action, "more silver" does not equal "works better."

Restated, higher concentrations do not necessarily kill more germs. If this wasn't true, we could just swallow silver coins and be done with it.

As an aside, the cost of silver as a raw material in structured silver is such a small fraction that it doesn't affect the choice of ppm at all. 10-30 ppm is chosen as the liquid's concentration because of its broad-spectrum efficacy.

If it were me I would take the ten parts per million product for everyday prevention and maintenance and save the 30 ppm silver for more severe medical crisis. In the laboratory 30 ppm silver destroys pathogens in a shorter period of time. The 30 ppm silver kills just as completely as 10 ppm silver but does so about 45 second faster than the 10 ppm.

Q: What is the shelf life?

A: Officially, two years. Given that it is a stable solution, it may be good for much longer than that.

Q: Does it need to be refrigerated?

A: No, room temperature is fine.

Q: Where is it made?

A: It is made in the United States under strict levels of quality control and GMP manufacturing standards.

Q: Who can take structured silver?

A: Anyone can take silver, but children under 75 pounds should take half the adult doses. And children younger than one should take one-third the normal adult dose. By the way, the normal adult dose of the structured silver liquid is two teaspoons twice a day.

Q: When is the best time to take it?

A: Take it at a time where you will not forget to take it. The best time to take it for daily prevention is two teaspoons twice a day (morning and night).

Q: Does structured silver affect my other medications, food, beverages, etc.?

A: No, it can be taken with anything except salt. The chloride ion binds with the silver and can neutralize some of the silver.

Q: Are there any contraindications using structured silver with any prescription products?

A: Don't mix structured silver with salt. The chloride ion binds with the silver and removes the silver's benefits. Beyond the neutralizing benefits of salt, there are no contraindications. If you are concerned about this, take the structured silver one hour before or after you take other medications or foods.

Q: Is it better to take structured silver with food or on an empty stomach?

A: If you take silver on an empty stomach there will be less salt to interfere with it. If you take it on an empty stomach you will also absorb the silver about 15 minutes faster than if you take it with food.

Q: Should structured silver be used daily or just when I have a problem?

A: Structured silver is designed to be used daily as a preventative. It can be taken two teaspoons twice a day as a liquid. It should be used twice a day or as needed as a gel. When a person has a more dramatic need they can double this dose, and in some severe cases people have successfully taken four ounces per day for up to two weeks.

Q: How does structured silver support immune function?

A: Structured silver benefits the immune system directly by moderately improving the number of immune cells that are capable of surveying for disease and destroying foreign pathogens. Structured silver benefits the immune system indirectly by killing the bacteria and viruses the cause disease, thus reducing the workload from an already overworked immune system and allowing the immune system to refocus its energies and recharge.

Q: How long does structured silver stay in the body? Can it accumulate over time?

A: Research suggests that 98% of the structured silver leaves the body by the next day. Argyria can occur when the silver stays in the body, but you would have to drink a ten times normal dose for decades (and none of it could leave your body) before you would begin to have symptoms of Argyria. It is the ionic and colloidal silver users that have too high concentrations of silver that cause Argyria.

Q: What is structured pH-balanced silver technology?

A: It is advanced scientific research and new product development specifically applied to structured pH-balanced (or alkaline) silver. The silver used in structured pH-balanced or alkaline silver technology is pure metallic silver and the term structured refers a chemical designation for something that is permanently suspended into the structure of water. Alkaline silver is a pure metallic silver permanently suspended in pure water and balanced with a slight alkaline pH of 7.5.

Q: What does structured pH-balanced silver do?

A: According to scientific reports structured silver has the ability to destroy bacteria, viruses, mold, yeast, and a limited number of parasites. It also can purify water.

Q: What health conditions does structured alkaline silver help with?

A: Structured alkaline silver could help with any disease that is caused by bacteria, viruses, yeast and some parasites, as long as the silver liquid or gel can come in contact with the pathogen for about 6 minutes.

I have seen it help with diseases inside the body as well as topically. I have seen it destroy hundreds of bacteria, both forms of viruses, yeasts and molds. The use must be creative to deliver the silver liquid or gel or aerosol to the site of the germ. Because the silver is water-soluble it is very safe and won't harm the good probiotic bacteria, but it won't pass through all tissues unless it is actively transported by the body or delivered in unique ways. Those are listed in the uses section of this book.

Q: How does structured silver work?

A: Structured silver destroys bacteria, virus and mold (yeast). These are the causes of disease. So silver destroys the cause of many diseases.

Silver works in numerous ways but we will focus on the most common mechanisms of action: As a silver oxide, viral disruption and resonance.

- As a silver oxide it will remove an electron from the bacterial membrane, thus rupturing the pathogen and killing it.
- As a viral disruption it can bind with the charged, incomplete genetic viral molecules, preventing viral replication, thus rendering the virus unable to duplicate itself.
- As a resonant frequency. This is a germicidal frequency which can destroy bacteria, viruses and mold, especially when it is alkaline.

Mechanism of Action
Structured alkaline silvers functions as a non-toxic internal or external disinfectant that is delivered to the site requiring disinfection (internal or external) via one or several of three separate delivery systems: liquid, topical gel and aerosolized.

The active ingredient is a nontoxic structured alkaline silver.

Structured alkaline silvers uses three primary mechanisms for action. Those mechanisms are I. Silver oxide II. Resonance III. Magnetic viral DNA disruption.

Mech. I – Silver Oxide – kills on contact with the bacteria by pulling one electron off the bacterial cell membrane, thereby rupturing the bacterial cell.

Mech. II – Resonance – the silver resonates at an antimicrobial frequency. Because it is small enough (a nanoparticle) to enter the host's cells, it transmits the resonant frequency without additional risk of exposure to the surrounding tissue, especially in an alkaline balance.

Mech. III – Magnetic Viral DNA Disruption – Viruses consist of a capsid that contains incomplete DNA segment0,s each containing a slight magnetic charge. The silver particle is engineered (structured) with a charge that inherently attracts the viral DNA and mechanically interferes with the ability of the Viral DNA to replicate. Note that because normal DNA contains a neutral magnetic charge, it remains unaffected by the charge of the structured alkaline silver.

By missing two electrons in the outer shell it can use one to bind with and remove a single electron from a bacteria and then recharge itself again and again. This means it has all the benefits of a colloid or ionic silver but is supercharged to a point that it can continue to remove electrons continuously, while colloids and ionic silvers can only inactivate one electron per silver particle.

All hospitals and labs that have constant germ exposure use germicidal lights that kill bacteria, viruses and germs simply by resonating at a frequency that destroys germs. This frequency is 910 terahertz. It is a similar frequency that the new structured silver resonates.

Q: Is structured silver safe?

A: Structured silver is produced in extremely low parts per million (5-40 ppm) and has never even been identified as a potential for problem in the water treatment plants or in the environment. This is significant because the EPA has a rating for toxic spills. This identifies the amount of a compound that would cause a toxic event. For instance, Clorox would qualify as a toxic event if 3 gallons were spilled. In contrast, the EPA would require a spill of 12.5 million gallons of silver liquid in order to be classified as a toxic event (5). This would require spilling the entire contents of 12.5 oil tankers at one time in one place without any other water to dilute it. There is no consumer or combination of consumers that store this much silver anywhere in the country.

An average water treatment plant treats about 30 to 70 million gallons of water a day and it would take a spill of about 7 tankers full of silver directly into the treatment water to bring the concentration to 1 part per million. This is still a very safe level for fish, and an impossible event to happen anywhere in the world.

Safety
Structured alkaline silver fulfills the definition of non-toxic, in that it passes through the body unchanged, which means it does not produce any harmful metabolites.

The CRC Handbook to Chemistry and Physics (sec 15 pg 8) states: "While silver is not considered to be toxic, most of its salts are poisonous." This is why alkaline silver containing only elemental silver and water is virtually devoid of toxicity. The only adverse event known for silver is Argyria, yet the EPA's lowest observed adverse event level (LOAEL) is given to silver. The EPA has determined that, administering one gram total elemental silver over a 2 year period presents no risk for developing Argyria.[59]

Safety

- Silver contains 0.00099% silver in distilled purified structured water.
- Argyria and nephrotoxicity are extremely unlikely to occur with a structured silver product due to the low concentration of contained silver. (EPA)
- A 16-oz bottle of silver contains micrograms of silver, which is thousands of times less than 1 gram.
- If a spill occurred it would take 12,500,000 gallons of silver to be considered by the EPA as a "reportable spill".
- According to EPA Guidelines, the oral consumption of small amounts of silver in water on a daily basis, poses NO significant risk.
- Silver would not be considered toxic at a dose of 5 mg/kg in mice and 2, 16-oz bottles of structured alkaline silver 10 ppm (NAMSA)
- Elemental silver is not considered a hazardous metal (Merck Index).

The Merck Index reports the following about silver:

It is a metal that does not accumulate in the fats and is the only metal that is not considered to be a heavy metal because it does not produce heavy metal poisoning.[60]

According to IRIS report Silver is:

- Non-toxic at 5000 mg/kg body weight.[61]
- 90%-99% leaves the body by the next day.
- Safe and non-toxic (it would take a spill of over 12 million gallons to be considered a reportable spill.[62]

Q: How much silver should I take?

A: Most people will want to take two teaspoons twice a day; if they get sick they will want to take two tablespoons twice a day. Consult this book, in the "Uses" section, for hundreds of more successful recommendations.

Q: Will I turn blue when I take structured alkaline silver?

A: Nobody has turned blue from the new structured alkaline silver. Ionic and colloidal silvers of the past have caused the blue-man coloring because they use a different and much higher concentration of silver in an acidic salt form of silver. You would have to drink 8 ounces a day every day for decades to turn blue with structured silver. So stay with the suggestions on the bottle and outlined in this book.

Q: Does it really matter to have alkaline of pH-balanced silver?

A: Yes, because the body heals best in alkaline balance. Acids make the healing process difficult and promote scarring. Alkaline silver is a terrific advancement in healthy silver.

Q: How long has silver been used to improve health benefits?

A: About 1000 years. Silver has been used as medicine and preservatives by many cultures throughout history. Greeks used silver vessels for water purification. Pioneers trekking across the west used it to keep their water safe and prevent dysentery, colds and flu. They actually put silver dollars in their milk containers and wooden water casks to retard the growth of bacteria. Settlers in the Australian outback suspend silverware in their water tanks to retard spoilage.

Q: Why is it important to have structured silver water?

A: Structured water is essential to keep the contaminants out of the silver. Most silver is contaminated and acidic and the silver is coated with a protein or contaminant coating. By using the structured water you reduce these problems and have a more pure, alkaline, better-absorbed silver, promoting the healing process without the acidic contaminated waters of most other silvers.

Q: Why use silver as a liquid; can't I just wear a silver necklace or ring?

A: Silver resonates at very effective frequency to destroy the causes of disease, bacteria, viruses, and yeast. Jewelry has some benefits that are good, but it is not the same, nor is it as comprehensive as the structured alkaline silver liquid or gel that can enter the cells.

Q: Is structured alkaline silver a nutritional supplement, food, drug or something else?

A: Structured alkaline silver is a nutritional supplement that passes through the body unchanged. It is a liquid or gel. This is important because it could also be considered to be a medical device, as it passes through the body unchanged. Silver has benefits that are scientifically proven while safe enough to be a food supplement.

Nelson Labs Reports

Alkaline structured silver destroyed more pathogens (MRSA) than any other form of silver tested by a factor of 1.4 log. This means there were about 1.4 million bacteria still alive in the other silver dishes when there was complete death of the bacteria in the pH-balanced alkaline silver. This helps demonstrate how the alkalinity contributes to pathogenic cell destruction and prevention of grow-back. In five minutes alkaline silver will effectively destroy more pathogens than any other silver tested.[63]

Appendix A

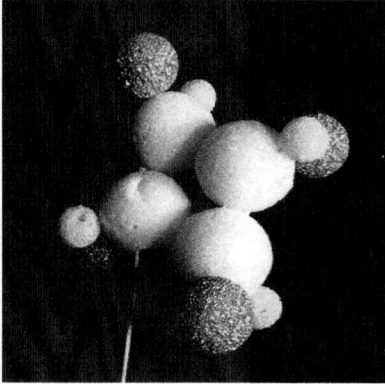

Structured Silver (Ag_4O_4, Ag_4O_4, Ag_4O_4, Ag_4O_4) Molecule

Silver (Ag_4O_4, Ag_4O_4, Ag_4O_4, Ag_4O_4) are structured water where four atoms of silver are permanently bonded into a tetrahedral crystalline structure with water and functions as a silver II oxide. There are four atoms of silver bound to the tetrahedral water crystal where two of the silver atoms are monovalent and the other two silver atoms are trivalent. The monovalent silver atoms are missing one electron in their valence while the trivalent silver atoms are missing three electrons in their outer valence shell. This is identified as a di-electro-magnet because there are two separate charges (energy states) on the same molecule. The silver atoms share a high energy particle that passes at very high speed between the monovalent and the trivalent silver atoms, producing a molecule that functions as if it were bi-valent (labeled as a silver II oxide). This is because the overall charge of the Ag_4O_4 molecule functions as if it were missing two electrons, when in reality half the molecule is monovalent and the other half of the molecule is trivalent. The structured alkaline silver molecule has been manufactured using a method that transfers a specific energy which produces a structured molecule with two high-energy particles that travel back and forth so fast that it vibrates between these two states. This vibration is produced by the rapid change from a silver I state to a silver III state and results in a molecular plasma that is sending out or resonating a frequency that has been identified as having antimicrobial activity. It should also be noted that the structure of this silver plasma-like molecule selectively binds to rapidly replicating bacteria and yeast due to the fact that these pathogens produce nitrogen and sulfur, which are expressed as a residue on the surface of the pathogen, resulting in cell signals that are chemically different that normal cells.

Ag_4O_4 is a di-electro-magnetic semiconductor that resonates at an antimicrobial frequency or frequencies. There are four water (H_2O) molecules that hold a structure for the four silver atoms to permanently attach.

References:

1. Clear Springs Press, Colloidal Silver.
2. Fox, C.J. Jr., 1968. Silver sulfadiazine, a new topical therapy for Pseudomonas burns. Arch. Surg. 96:184–188.
3. Fox, C. J., 1969. Control of Pseudomonas infection in burns by Silver Sulfadiazine. Surg. Gynecol. Obstet. 128:1021–1026.
4. IRIS Report, 2005.
5. EPA Report and Guidelines #D011.
6. U.S House International Relations Committee, 2005. Written testimony on Black Mold and MRSA.
7. U.S House International Relations Committee, 2005. Written testimony on Black Mold and MRSA.
8. EPA, Reregistration Eligibility Document (RED). Office of Prevention Pesticides and Toxic Substances (H-7508W). EPP 738-R-93-005 June 1993.
9. IRIS Report, 2005.
10. The Merck Manual, 1999. Section 226 Nephropathy.
11. Merck Index., 1999. Silver. 1:645. 13. IRIS Report, 200516. EPA report and guidelines #D011.
12. Nichols, J., Acute Oral Toxicity Study in the Rat, NAMSA, 2009. Oral Ingestion of High Doses of Silver Demonstrates No Toxicity In Rats.
13. Duan, L, et al. "Rapid and simultaneous detection of human hepatitis B virus and hepa-titis C virus antibodies based on a protein chip assay using nanogold immunological am-plification and silver staining method." BMC Infect Dis., 2005 Jul 6;5:53.
14. Chang, AL, et al. "A case of argyria after colloidal silver ingestion." J Cutan Pathol. 2006 Dec;33(12):809–11.
15. Arch Otoolyryngol Head Neck Surg, Bartlett, JG, Froggatt, WIII, 1995, 121(4): p392-96.
16. Colloids in Biology and Medicine, Beckhold H., New York. D. Von Nostrand. 1919 pg 364-76.

17. The Body Electric, Electromagnetism and the foundation of life. Becker, R.O., Seldon, G., New York, Morrow, 1985.

18. Newsweek, Mar, 1994, pg 46-51, Begley, S.

19. Antimicrobial Agents and Chemotherapy, Berger, TJ, Antifungal Properties of Electrically Generated metallic Ions. 1976; (10) pg 856-60.

20. Antimicrobial Agents and Chemotherapy, 1976; (9): p357-58. Berger, TJ, Electrically Generated Silver Ions.

21. Surgical Forum, vol. 17, 1966, pg 76-78. Brentano, L., Antibacterial Efficacy of a Colloi-dal Silver.

22. Arch Surg., 1968(97): pg 716. Burke, JF., Bondoc, CC., Combined burn therapy utilizing immediate skin allographs and 0.5% silver nitrate.

23. Antimicrobial Agents Chemother., 1973; (4): pg 585-87. Carr, H., Wlodkowki, TJ. Silver Sulfadiazine: In Vitro Antibacterial Activity.

24. Journal of Infectious Disease., 1975; july, 132(1) pg 79-81. In vitro activity of silver sul-fadiazine against Herpesvirus Hominus.

25. Antimicrobial Agents and Chemotherapy., 1975-8):pg 677-78. Chang, TW, Weinstein, L., Prevention of Herpes Keratoconjunctivitis in Rabbits by silver sulfadiazine.

26. British Journal of Medicine., 1923: Feb 17:p273-277. Clark, A., The properties of certain colloidal preparations of metals.

27. Cambridge University Press., 1989, Crosby, A., The forgotten pandemic: The influenza pandemic of 1918.

28. Lancet, 1912:jan 13, Duhamel, B., Electric Metal Colloids and Their Therapeutical Appli-cations.

29. Elsevier Science Pub., 1986, vol 2: pg 521-31. Fowler, B., Nordberg, G., "Silver" in the handbook on the toxicology of Metals.

30. The Coming Plague., Newly emerging diseases in a world out of balance, Garrett, L., New York. Penguin. 1995, p.413.

31. Biochem Biophysics Res. Comm., 1992: (189): p 1444-49. Hussain, S., Cystein Protects Na, K-ATPase and isolated human lymphocytes form silver toxicity.

32. Annul Rev Med., 1996, 47: p 169-79. Jacoby GA. Antimicrobial-resistant pathogens in the 1900's.

33. Ayurveda: The Science of Self-Healing: A practical guide. Santa Fe. Lotus Press. 1984.

34. Pediatr Clin North Am. 1995; 42(3):649-664. Longworth, DL., Drug resistant malaria in children and travelers.

35. Lancet. 1912, Feb 3. MacLeod, CE, Electric Metallic Colloids and Their Therapeutical Applications.

36. Science Digest. 1978: mar p 57-60. Powell,J., Silver our Mightiest Germ Fighter.

37. The British Journal of Medicine. 1913; nov: p 83. Searle, AB., The use of colloids in health and disease.

38. Proc. Nat Acad of Science USA, 1994; 91 (7): p 2420-27. Swartz, MN., Hospital acquired infections: diseases with increasingly limited therapies.

39. CRC Critical Review Environmental Control. 1989: (18): p295-315. Thurman, R., Gerba, C., The molecular mechanisms of copper and silver ion disinfection of bacteria and vi-ruses.

40. Am Journal of Obstetrics. 1916: jan: p 136-141.Van Amber Brown, G., Colloidal silver in sepsis.

41. Lancet. 1973; Sep 29: p 739-40.Wlodkowski, T., Rosenkranz, H., Antifungal activity of silver sulfadiazine.

42. EPA, regulation on Silver. (US EPA Silver; CASRN 7440-22-4 1996).

43. EPA, Reregistration Eligibility Document (RED). Office of Prevention Pesticides and Toxic Substances (H-7508W). EPP 738-R-93-005 June 1993).

44. Pedersen, G., Journal of the Society of Healing Outcomes, 2006. Effect of prophylactic treatment with Silver Sol Solutions on an Avian Influenza A (H5N1) Virus Infection in Mice.

45. Bush RM, Fitch WM, Bender CA, Cox NJ. Positive selection on the H3 hemagglutinin gene of human influenza virus A. Mol Biol Evol. 1999;16:1457–1465.

46. Townsend Letters for Doctors, May 2006.

47. Am Acad Environmental Medicine, 2003.

48. Bull Cancer, 2006.

49. Eur. Neurology, 2002.

50. J. Biol Regul Homeost Agents, 2005.

51. Pediatrics, 2005.

52. J Support Oncology, 2005.

53. Bone Marrow Transplant, 2005.

54. Cancer, 2005.

55. Medicine, 2005.

56. Becker, 1995.

57. Antelman, MS. 2000.

58. JAMA, Oct. 2007.

59. U.S. EPA Silver; CASRN 7440-22-4 1996.

60. Merck Index., 1999. Silver. 1:645.

61. IRIS Report, 2005.

62. Merck Index., 1999. Silver. 1:645. 13. IRIS Report, 200516. EPA report and guidelines #D011.

63. Nelson Labs. Alkaline silver outperforms other forms of silver by log 1.4.

To Order Additional Copies Please Call: 801.923.4352 or visit Amazon.com, DrGoPed.com or SilverHealthInstitute.com.

The statements, research and any claims implied or made in this book do not refer to any one specific product rather structured silver products as a whole. NONE OF THE STATEMENTS IN THIS BOOK HAVE BEEN REVIEWED BY THE FDA. Consult your personal care provider before beginning or changing any supplemental or prescription regimen.

Index

Printed in Great Britain
by Amazon